MANUAL OF PAEDIATRIC GASTRO-ENTEROLOGY AND NUTRITION

Second Edition

John H Tripp BSc MD FRCP

Senior Lecturer in Child Health
Postgraduate Medical School
University of Exeter
Exeter, UK

David C A Candy MSc MD FRCP

Professor of Child Health
King's College School of Medicine and Dentistry
London, UK

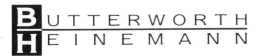

Butterworth-Heinemann Ltd
Linacre House, Jordan Hill, Oxford OX2 8DP

 PART OF REED INTERNATIONAL BOOKS

OXFORD   LONDON   BOSTON
MUNICH   NEW DELHI   SINGAPORE   SYDNEY
TOKYO   TORONTO   WELLINGTON

First published by Churchill Livingstone 1985
Second edition published by Butterworth-Heinemann 1992

© Butterworth-Heinemann Ltd, 1992

British Library Cataloguing in Publication Data
Manual of paediatric gastroenterology and nutrition. – 2nd ed.
  I. Tripp, John H.   II. Candy, David C. A.
  618.92

ISBN 0 7506 1325 4

Library of Congress Cataloguing in Publication Data
Tripp, John H.
    Manual of paediatric gastroenterology and nutrition/John H.
  Tripp, David C. A. Candy. — 2nd ed.
      p.   cm.
  Rev. ed. of: Manual of pediatric gastroenterology, 1985.
  Includes index.
  ISBN 0 7506 1325 4
  1. Pediatric gastroenterology—Handbooks, manuals, etc.
I. Candy, David C. A.   II. Tripp, John H. Manual of pediatric
gastroenterology.   III. Title.
  [DNLM: 1. Gastrointestinal Diseases—in infancy & childhood—
handbooks.   WS 39 T836ma]
RJ446.T75   1991
618.92'33—dc20
DNLM/DLC
for Library of Congress   91-34007
                                                          CIP

Composition by Genesis Typesetting, Laser Quay, Rochester, Kent
Printed and bound in Great Britain by Redwood Press Limited,
Melksham, Wiltshire

MANUAL OF PAEDIATRIC
GASTROENTEROLOGY AND NUTRITION

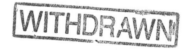

CONTENTS

PREFACE TO THE FIRST EDITION

Acute diarrhoea and its consequences of malnutrition, growth failure and subsequent infection continues to be the major cause of infant deaths in the world. Effective management in the Third World is a paramount activity of the World Health Organisation for the eighties.

In industrialised countries severe organic gastrointestinal problems stretch diagnostic, supportive and curative medical resources while functional disorders of the gastrointestinal tract remain ill-understood and often poorly managed. Some of the disorders presenting major challenges are so rare that consultant paediatricians see less than one new case per year (e.g. Crohn's disease) while others, so common, (e.g. constipation) that they are a burden to many family doctors.

The book's structure is problem-orientated and where possible this pattern continues within chapters. Our intention is to produce a book useful for practising doctors at work as well as to present material in an easily assimilated form for learning. We consider the telegraphic style of text makes the book particularly 'usable'. In listing points indicating clinical importance, clinical presentation, and so on, numbers have deliberately been omitted to avoid misunderstanding.

Our aim has been to provide a practical handbook for paediatricians but we hope it will be useful to paediatric surgeons, family practitioners and hospital and community nurses.

Exeter　　　　　　　　　　　　　　　　　　　　　　　J. H. Tripp
Birmingham　　　　　　　　　　　　　　　　　　　D. C. A. Candy
1985

PREFACE TO THE SECOND EDITION

— Reactions to first edition
  - We were gratified by generally good response
  - From reviewers
  - From our friends and colleagues
— We are therefore committed to this style of writing!

— This book reflects the personal practice of the authors
  - Not all our practice can be supported by original scientific articles
  - We have made no attempt to reference even contentious issues
  - It is not intended to replace standard texts but to be a 'bench book'
  - We believe its unique style lends itself to this use
— We are delighted to welcome two expert contributors
  - Dr Ian W. Booth a paediatric gastroenterologist who is responsible for nutritional care at the Birmingham Children's Hospital
  - Professor Stuart Tanner a paediatric gastroenterologist with a long-standing interest in liver disease of childhood both in the UK and Far East

Exeter
London
1991

J. H. Tripp
D. C. A. Candy

ACKNOWLEDGEMENTS

We sincerely record our gratitude to those who have enhanced our understanding of paediatrics and gastroenterology. We were helped enormously by the late Professor John Harries and also by Professor O. H. Wolff, Professor A. S. McNeish and Dr B. A. Wharton. The editors are delighted to welcome our two new contributors (Ian Booth and Stuart Tanner) who have enhanced our previous material enormously by their contributions. We are grateful to a number of people who have reviewed parts of the text for us, including: Dr Christopher Ellis, Consultant, Department of Communicable and Tropical Diseases, University of Birmingham; Miss Lucinda Henry, now dietitian at the Birmingham Children's Hospital; Anita McDonald, Dietitian, Birmingham Children's Hospital; Patrick Ball, Pharmacist at Birmingham Children's Hospital; Dr Sean Devane, King's College Hospital; and Dr Stephan Strobel, Hospital for Sick Children, Great Ormond Street.

We are most grateful to Sylvia Hull who first suggested the book and has enabled us to produce a further edition. We would like to express our thanks to Mrs Ann Hoskins and Miss Debbie Perry for providing us with a software manuscript that could be handled directly by the typesetters.

CONTRIBUTORS

Nutrition
Dr Ian W. Booth, Senior Lecturer in Child Health, Birmingham Children's
Hospital, Francis Road, Birmingham B16 8ET, UK

Hepatology
Professor Stuart Tanner, Professor of Paediatrics, Children's Hospital,
Western Bank, Sheffield S10 2TH, UK

1 NEONATAL GASTROINTESTINAL EMERGENCIES AND SURGERY

GENERAL ISSUES

Presentation

Obvious external anomaly
- Exomphalos (p. 3)
- Anal atresia (p. 14)
- Ectopia vesicae (not discussed)

Respiratory difficulty
- Diaphragmatic hernia (p. 4)
- Tracheo-oesophageal fistula (TOF)/atresia (p. 5)

Intestinal obstructive symptoms
- Vomiting (almost invariably bile stained)
- Abdominal distension
- Early onset suggests high lesion
  - Duodenal atresia (p. 8)
  - Jejunal atresia (p. 9)
  - Malrotation/volvulus (p. 10)
  - Duplication cysts (p. 7)
- 2nd day of life suggests midgut obstruction
  - Ileal atresia (p. 9)
  - Meconium ileus (p. 11)
  - Milk plug syndrome (p. 12)
  - Functional obstruction (p. 15)
  - Pseudo-obstruction (p. 16)
- Later onset suggests low or partial obstruction
  - Hirschsprung's (p. 12)
  - Anal atresia (p. 14)
  - Necrotising enterocolitis (p. 16)
  - Duodenal web (p. 8)

Bile stained vomiting
- Should always be regarded as probably pathological
  - Strongly suggests obstruction even if intermittent, e.g. partial volvulus

- • Also occurs in sick newborns prior to obstruction, e.g. necrotising enterocolitis
- — Duodenogastric reflux is not uncommon in small preterm infants
  - • Fluid is usually yellow rather than green

Blood in stools
- — Maternal
- — Necrotising enterocolitis (p. 16)
- — Infarction due to volvulus etc. (p. 10), asphyxia

Diarrhoea
- — Necrotising enterocolitis (p. 16)
- — Hirschsprung's enterocolitis (p. 12)
- — Inborn errors of absorption of electrolytes (p. 65) or carbohydrate (p. 63)

Emergency management, preoperative care

Preoperative assessment
- — Temperature
- — Hydration and biochemical status (electrolytes, creatinine, blood glucose, Ca^{2+})
- — Circulatory status
- — Respiratory status

Evaluation and assessment
- — Is it a real emergency? e.g. diaphragmatic hernia presenting at less than 12 h of age
- — Will delay enable fuller assessment, and more appropriate elective surgery or referral?
- — Are there other major congenital abnormalities? e.g. Down syndrome, cardiovascular malformation

Preparation for operation/transfer (general)
- — Pass nasogastric tube and leave on open drainage
- — Correct hypothermia, biochemical abnormality
- — Give vitamin K_1 (phytomenadione) 1 mg IM
- — Obtain 10 ml of maternal blood and group infant
- — Obtain signed parental consent after adequate explanation of aims and possible results of surgery

Transfer
- — Try and arrange transfer of mother with infant if possible
- — Ensure that mother sees/holds infant
- — Obtain 'Polaroid' photograph
- — Put the child to the breast if possible (not if TOF) and establish lactation by expression
- — Provide referral centre with adequate history and data
  - • Family and social history
  - • Obstetric history, delivery data, birthweight

- Record of observations such as passage of urine and/or meconium
- Results of investigations
  NB Microbiology results received after transfer must be forwarded
- Is baptism requested/required?
- Record of any treatment given (e.g. antibiotics)
— Send X-rays and clinical/nursing notes

SPECIFIC CONDITIONS

Exomphalos

— Any protrusion at the umbilicus (strictly excludes gastroschisis, but included here with omphalocoele and hernia in the cord)

Incidence

— 1 in 10 000 live births

Associated disorders

— Meckel's diverticulum
— Intestinal atresias
— Malrotation
— Beckwith syndrome (+ hypoglycaemia and macrosomia)

Hernia into the cord

— Persistence of the normal fetal umbilical hernia
— No abdominal wall defect
— Surgical repair usually straightforward
  NB Small herniae may be trapped in cord clamp leading to perforation

Omphalocoele

— Cord hernia with muscular defect in abdominal wall at umbilicus
— Large defects may contain other viscera, e.g. liver, bladder
— Ruptured exomphalos usually worst prognosis of any for gut function
— Small defects closed with skin flaps
— Large defects managed as gastroschisis

Gastroschisis

— Defect in abdominal wall, not at umbilicus
— Usually to right of midline
— No covering of amnion over viscera

Management

— Primary closure is achieved if possible
NB Replacement of gut in a small abdominal cavity will splint diaphragm and embarrass respiration
— Two-stage procedure
  • Viscera covered with sac (e.g. Silastic, Prolene) sutured around edge of lesion, returning as much as possible to abdominal cavity
  • Gradual reduction in size of sac over following weeks
  • External gut functions very poorly; prolonged intravenous nutrition is often required
— Stenoses not visible at operation may complicate recovery or present later

Diaphragmatic hernia (and eventration of diaphragm)

Aetiology

— Failure of pleuroperitoneal canal (foramen of Bochdalek) to close
— Commoner on the left side
— Eventration due to weak or absent diaphragmatic muscle, produces identical clinical picture

Incidence

— 1 in 2000 births

Clinical features

— Abdominal organs displaced into thorax
— Compressed lung hypoplastic

Presentation

— Acute presentation (less than 12 h poorer prognosis because of lung hypoplasia)
  • Increasing respiratory distress
  • Displacement of heart usually to right
  • Scaphoid abdomen
  • Dull percussion and decreased air entry on affected side
— Subacute presentation
  • Vomiting, feeding difficulty, constipation
  • Dyspnoea
— Incidental finding on X-ray

Diagnosis

— Clinical features as above
— Chest X-ray shows 'cystic' appearance of multiple loops of air-filled bowel in the thorax
  • Differential diagnosis of radiograph includes pneumomediastinum, cystic lung malformation, infection

Management

— Erect posture
— Avoid mask ventilation or continuous positive airways pressure

- Intermittent positive pressure ventilation via endotracheal tube
— Deflation and continuous drainage of stomach with nasogastric tube
— Surgical correction after stabilisation

Prognosis

— Immediate: dependent on prompt diagnosis and appropriate management
— Long term: determined by degree of pulmonary hypoplasia

Oesophageal atresia and tracheo-oesophageal fistula

Aetiology

— Failure of separation of trachea and oesophagus in fourth week of gestation
— (Figure 1.1 shows different anatomical variants)

Incidence

— 1 in 3000 live births in UK
— Associated major anomaly in 50%

Presentation

— Maternal polyhydramnios in 25% (not H type)
— Drooling 'mucousy' infants
  NB This should suggest the diagnosis before the first feed
— Aspiration of first mouthful of feed: regurgitation, cough, cyanosis, apnoea
— Regurgitation of gastric contents to trachea with pneumonitis (not type a or b)
— No air below diaphragm on X-ray (type a or b)
— Subacute presentation (H type) with feeding problems: choking, coughing, respiratory distress, recurrent chest infections, abdominal distension

Diagnosis

— Whenever there is any clinical suspicion, before giving the first feed
— Pass wide-bore (to prevent kinking) orogastric tube into oesophagus
— If it 'arrests' before reaching stomach
  - Aspirate and inject a little air
  - X-ray chest

H-type

— Occurs anywhere between cricoid and bifurcation of trachea
— Usually slopes upward from oesophagus to trachea
— May be multiple
— Requires expert paediatric radiology and endoscopy to exclude
  - Repeated examinations may be required

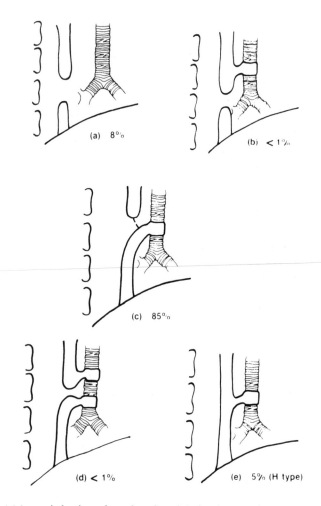

Figure 1.1 Anatomical variants of oesophageal atresia and tracheo-oesophageal fistula

Management

Emergency

— Directed towards prevention of aspiration and pneumonitis
- Nurse sitting upright (or prone in incubator)
- Use Replogle tube to keep upper oesophageal pouch empty by continuous suction
- Culture tracheal aspirate and blood and start broad spectrum antibiotic if aspiration has occurred

— Check blood glucose and treat if necessary

— Transfer to paediatric surgical unit

Surgical
- Primary oesophageal anastomosis and closure of fistula possible in 75%
  - Feed via transanastomotic nasojejunal tube if Lipiodol swallow is normal at 5 days after operation
- If primary anastomosis impossible:
  - Fistula divided
  - Feeding gastrostomy
  - Usually upper pouch oesophagostomy to allow drainage and sham feeding
  - Later (e.g. 1 year or 9 kg) secondary anastomosis or alternative surgery, e.g. colon transplant

Complications

Associations
- Look for features of VATER association
  - Vertebral anomalies
  - Ventriculoseptal defects
  - Anal atresia
  - Tracheo-oesophageal fistula
  - Radial dysplasia
  - Renal anomaly

Postoperative
- Breakdown of anastomosis
- Erosion of posterior wall of trachea – recurrence as H Type fistula
- Mediastinitis, pneumothorax, pyothorax

Late
- Swallowing difficulties
  - 'Obstruction' with solids
  - Recurrent aspiration

Prognosis
- 65–90% survival in different series
  - Most mortality occurs in those with associated malformations

Duplications

Pathology
- All occur on the mesenteric border of the normal gut
  - They often share the same outer muscle layer
  - May be entirely separate and blind ending, or communicate at both ends with normal gut
  - May be cystic or tubular in type

Associations
- Thoracic with anterior spina bifida
  - May track down through the diaphragm and communicate with abdominal viscera

— Tubular with vertebral abnormalities including hemi- and split vertebrae as the split notochord syndrome

Presenting features
— Neonatal respiratory distress
— Intestinal obstruction
— Volvulus
— Abdominal distension
— Abdominal mass
— Cystic appearance or space occupying lesion on chest X-ray
— Bleeding from heterotopic gastric mucosa
— Blind loop syndrome
— Meningitis from anterior spina bifida

Diagnosis
— Straight X-ray showing dense mass or fluid level
— Contrast studies showing stretching of intestine over the lesion and possibly filling of communicating lesions

Surgery
— Small or cystic duplication often excised with the adjacent normal gut because of shared blood supply
— Tubular duplications managed by stripping the mucosa from inside the duplication, leaving serosa and muscle in situ to avoid lengthy resections of normal intestine

SMALL INTESTINE OBSTRUCTION

Duodenal atresia

Aetiology of duodenal obstruction
— Extrinsic
  • Malrotation (Ladd's bands)
  • Volvulus
— Intrinsic
  • Atresia
  • Stenosis
  • Diaphragm

Incidence
— 1 per 5000 live births in UK
— Commonest site is second part of duodenum
  • May be associated with annular pancreas
— Other major anomaly is common
  • 30% of duodenal atresia is associated with Down syndrome

Clinical features
— Maternal polyhydramnios
— Vomiting

- Usually within 24 hours
- Usually bile stained as lesion at second part or beyond

Diagnosis
— Inject 5–10 ml of air down nasogastric tube
— Erect abdominal X-ray
  - Characteristic double bubble of fluid levels with air above in stomach and duodenal cap
  - Distension of stomach and proximal duodenum
  - No air in rest of gastrointestinal tract

Management

Emergency
— Aspirate stomach contents with adequate bore tube and leave on free drainage with hourly aspiration
— Correction of fluid and electrolyte deficit if necessary. (Use saline to correct alkalosis)

Surgery
— Careful examination of the rest of the gastrointestinal tract
— Transanastomotic feeding tube (fine-bore Silicone)
— Wide-bore nasogastric tube ensures adequate gastric drainage
— Parental nutrition is often required for a period (see p. 153)

Prognosis
— Similar to, though slightly better than, oesophageal atresia

Jejunal and ileal atresias

Incidence
— 1 in 6000 live births in UK
— Single or multiple
— Often associated with evidence of localised meconium peritonitis

Clinical features
— Maternal polyhydramnios only in proximal lesions
— Vomiting occurs early with proximal lesions
— Abdominal distension later and more severe in distal lesions
— Delay in passage of meconium
— Rectal washout may reveal white plugs only

Diagnosis
— Erect X-ray of abdomen
  - Small bowel fluid levels
  - Grossly distended segment, immediately proximal to atresia
  - No gas in rectum
— Supine X-ray of abdomen
  - May show speckled calcification of meconium peritonitis

Management
— As for duodenal atresia
— Transanastomotic tube may not be practical if atresia is distal

— Tapering of dilated segment by removing a 'tuck' may be desirable to aid effective peristalsis

— Record length and type of remaining small intestine

— Specific therapy required if terminal ileum has been resected (see under Short gut syndrome, p. 168)

Prognosis

— Survival over 85%

— High mortality with
  - Multiple atresias
  - Massive resection
  - Associated anomalies

Malrotation and small intestine volvulus

Aetiology

— Disordered embryogenesis between 6th and 16th week
  - Failure of rotation of caecum around small intestine
  - Failure of fusion of caecal mesentery with parietal peritoneum
  - Ladd's bands from posterior abdominal wall and gall bladder across the second part of the duodenum
  - Leaves large bowel on left side of abdomen and small intestine on the right
  - Small intestine has a narrow pedicle and can rotate on this to produce volvulus

Clinical features

— Duodenal obstruction by Ladd's bands

— Partial, intermittent or complete duodenal or small intestinal obstruction due to volvulus
  - Food refusal
  - Blood stained vomiting
  - Abdominal distension
  - Abdominal pain
  - Passage of blood in faeces

— Partial obstruction with malabsorption

Diagnosis

Acute presentation

— See diagnosis of duodenal obstruction

— Dilated, gas-filled loops in centre of abdomen in volvulus

Intermittent

— Barium follow through
  - May show duodenal obstruction
  - Characteristic S-shaped duodenum turning down or right at 3rd part to small bowel which is mostly on the right

— Barium enema
  - Caecum in midline or left hypochondrium
  - Large bowel mostly on the left

Management

— Volvulus is a surgical emergency
   NB A massive infarction and resection may be the result of delay in diagnosis or surgery
— Surgery
   • Always indicated if volvulus suspected
   • May not need to be done as an emergency if no signs of obstruction/strangulation
   • Division of Ladd's bands
   • Possible lengthening of small bowel mesentery
   • Consider fixation of bowel to abdominal wall
   • Some surgeons carry out routine appendicectomy
— Strangulation
   • Frankly infarcted gut is resected
   • Probable double barrelled enterostomies
   • Consider reopening abdomen in 24 hours to re-examine areas of doubtful viability

Meconium ileus

Aetiology

— Intestinal obstruction due to impaction of viscid meconium
— Usually due to cystic fibrosis
— Presenting feature of 5–10% of cystic fibrosis
— Can occur in absence of cystic fibrosis (5% of cases)

Clinical features

— Failure to pass meconium
— Abdominal distension
— Visible and palpable loops of bowel
— Bile stained vomiting

Diagnosis

— Erect X-ray of abdomen
   • Paucity of fluid levels
   • Granular appearance of bowel contents
   • Possible calcification of meconium peritonitis
— Gastrografin (Schering) enema is diagnostic; the contrast outlining the meconium

Management

— Detergent action of Gastrografin may relieve obstruction
— May be used if
   • No evidence of perforation
   • General condition and hydration satisfactory
   • Facilities for immediate operation available
   NB Hyperosmolar solution dehydrates infant if retained
   NB Excessive hydrostatic pressure may perforate gut
— Acetyl cysteine orally (5 ml of 10% solution) every 8 hours and by enema may relieve the obstruction

— Surgery (if medical management fails)
  • Multiple enterotomies may be required if the viscid material is to be removed
  • A Bishop–Koop ileostomy provides safety valve while the distal meconium clears itself
  • Ileostomy closed when infant is thriving
— Cystic fibrosis should be excluded
  • Faecal chymotrypsin probably the best test
  • Plasma immunoreactive trypsin also useful
  • Later sweat test
  • Screen siblings if positive

Meconium plug

— A term normally applied to a rectal meconium plug common in preterm infants
— Simple removal with a washout may produce a 10–15 cm 'plug' followed by copious meconium
— May be presenting feature of meconium ileus or Hirschsprung's (see p. 11)

Milk plug (bolus) obstruction

— Rare in breast-fed infants
— Commoner with unmodified formulae

Clinical features

— Features of small intestinal obstruction
  • Mass in right iliac fossa
  • Usually at 5–10 days of age
  • Perforation may occur

Diagnosis

— Erect abdominal X-ray shows dilated loops and fluid levels
— Gastrografin enema may be diagnostic and curative as in meconium ileus

Management

— As for meconium ileus
  • Bolus can usually be broken up at laparotomy
  • Ileostomy rarely required

LARGE INTESTINAL OBSTRUCTION

Hirschsprung's disease

Aetiology

— Absence of ganglion cells in intramuscular and submucous plexuses

- Involves a variable length of intestine from anus extending proximally
- Ultra-long segment may be familial/genetic

Clinical features
Neonatal
— Failure to pass meconium
- 10% of normal infants do not in first 24 h and 2% do not pass in first 48 h
— Signs of large bowel obstruction
- Abdominal distension (gross, especially flanks)
- Vomiting (late, possibly faeculant)
— Rectum empty
— Removal of finger may be associated with a 'spurt' of meconium or faeces (toothpaste sign)

Later
— Chronic constipation dating from birth
— Abdominal distension
— Failure to thrive

Diagnosis

Rectal biopsy
— Suction biopsies at 2 and 5 cm
- Stained for ganglion cells (absent in Hirschsprung's)
- Stained for cholinesterase (increased in nerve fibres in Hirschsprung's)
- Most reliable diagnostic test

Anorectal manometry
— Anal pressures measured during rectal distension by a fluid-filled balloon
- Normal relaxation of internal sphincter does not occur in Hirschsprung's
- May detect 'ultra-short segment' disease
- Very reliable in experienced hands

Contrast enema
— Shows characteristic 'funnel' or 'cone' of dilated normal bowel leading to the affected segment
- False positive and false negative results may be obtained (see also small left colon syndrome)
- May be useful for estimating length of affected segment preoperatively

Management
— Relief of obstruction by an enterostomy sited just proximal to aganglionic segment using frozen sections to establish site
— At 1 year, a bypass of aganglionic segment by
- Duhamel: end to side anastomosis behind rectum
- Swenson: pull through anal anastomosis

- Soave: resection, removal of anal mucosa and a pull through operation
— In older children, single stage operation is usual

Complications

Enterocolitis
— Acute
- May occur before or after neonatal surgery for Hirschsprung's disease
- Carries a high mortality
- Managed by relief of obstruction and as necrotising enterocolitis
— Subacute
- Some infants may present during the first year with diarrhoea and subacute enterocolitis due to Hirschsprung's disease

Faecal incontinence
— 70–90% achieve continence
— This may be delayed until adolescence
— Colostomy may be required in some patients

Colonic atresia

— Only one-twentieth as common as small intestinal atresia
— Presents later with signs of large bowel obstruction
— Management as for small bowel obstruction

Anal atresia

Types
— Classified as low, middle and high
— Atresia or stenosis

Low (infralevator)
— Intestine terminates below pelvic floor
— Effectively a covered anus
— Anal site marked by triangular skin tag
- Apex forwards at the anus
— There may be meconium staining in the skin
— Treatment is by excision of the cover
— Follow up dilatation is required

High (supralevator)
— Intestine terminates above the pelvic floor
— Either totally blind or with a fistula
- Fistula may be to bladder, vagina or skin
— Surgery
- Transverse colostomy
- Later (6–12 months) elective 'pull through'
NB Associated anomalies are common
— Complications after surgery as for Hirschsprung's)

Diagnosis
- Absent or blind ending anus on digital or soft tube probing
- Plain abdominal X-ray
  - In inverted position for gas to outline rectal pouch
  - With radio-opaque marker at position of anus
- Contrast medium enema or cystogram to demonstrate any fistulae

Surgical treatment
- Defunctioning colostomy initially
- Close associated rectovesical fistula early to prevent urinary tract infection
- Corrective operation at approximately 6 months
  - Anoplasty, anastomosis or excision of fistula depending on anatomy
  - Careful positioning of anus in relation to external anal sphincter
  - Preservation of anorectal sling and associated nerve supply

Complications
- Acute
  - Dehydration
  - Respiratory restriction due to severe abdominal distension
  - Aspiration pneumonia secondary to vomiting
- Late
  - Constipation from residual of anal stenosis/fibrosis
  - Faecal incontinence if internal anal sphincter zone is narrow

Prognosis
- Good prognosis for survival
- Depends on associated anomalies. NB VATER (p. 7)
- Faecal continence depends on:
  - Length of effective internal anal sphincter zone
  - Function of puborectalis sling
  - Avoidance of constipation and overflow incontinence

Functional obstruction and intestinal pseudo-obstruction
- Symptoms and signs of intestinal obstruction without anatomical or histological abnormality

Functional obstruction
- Often large bowel
- Occurs in
  - Infants of diabetic mothers
  - Sick preterm infants
  - Post gastroschisis repair
  - Idiopathic with apparently ineffective motility in segments of bowel
- May mimic Hirschsprung's
  - Hypoganglionosis has been described in some of the idiopathic cases

Intestinal pseudo-obstruction
— Specific inherited disorder
  • Chronic adynamic bowel syndrome
  • Dominantly inherited with variable penetrance
  • Poor prognosis
  • Contrast studies show proximal dilated gut
  • Adynamic segments
  • May require excision of affected segment if localised
— Urinary tract smooth muscle may be affected also
— May be the presenting feature of mucosal neuroma syndrome
  • Neurofibromatous malformation of lips and oral cavity
  • Massive nerve trunks on rectal biopsy
  • Alternating severe constipation and diarrhoea
  • Potential for medullary carcinoma of thyroid
  • Dominantly inherited

Necrotising enterocolitis

Incidence
— Probably tenfold variation between neonatal units
— Commoner in preterm and those receiving intensive care
— May be commoner after umbilical vessel catheterisation
— Breast feeding may protect
  • Hyperosmolar feeds commonly believed to increase incidence
Aetiology
— Occurs in 'outbreaks' and in some neonatal units very much more often than others
— Pathology resembles a necrotic enteritis, 'pigbel' caused by *Clostridium welchii* occurring in Papua New Guinea
— Infectious agent is probably implicated in outbreaks
— Pathological appearances suggest that mucosal ischaemia plays a role in pathogenesis
  • Supported by the fact that predisposing causes may lead to hypoxic injury to the gut
— Colon and ileum involved more often than jejunum
Presentation
— Frequently presents with non-specific clinical deterioration in newborn who is also frequently preterm and/or ventilated
  • Apnoeas and bradycardias
  • Hypothermia
  • Hyponatraemia
  • Low platelets, disseminated intravascular coagulation
  • Signs of infection
— Gastrointestinal (classical)
  • Bile stained vomiting
  • Blood stained stools

- Tender distended abdomen
- Reddened or even oedematous abdominal wall

Radiology

— Fixed dilated air-filled loops (often in splenic flexure area)
— Bubbly appearance of faecal shadows
— Thickened bowel wall
— Intramural gas
— Evidence of perforation with intraperitoneal gas

Management

— Rapid progress of symptoms and signs suggests poor prognosis

Conservative

— Appropriate for all cases unless there is evidence of perforation
— Remove nasojejunal tube if present (leave nasogastric tube only)
— Oral feeds stopped completely or reduced to 0.5 ml/kg/hour of expressed breast milk if no ileus
— Correction of anaemia, hypovolaemia (plasma), fluid and electrolyte balance
— Parenteral nutrition
— Systemic antibiotics (broad spectrum and metronidazole)
— Treatment of coagulopathy with fresh frozen plasma or exchange transfusion with fresh blood as indicated
— 12 hourly erect (or decubitius) X-rays to detect perforation
— Surgery may also be considered after initial acute stage if obstructive symptoms persist or develop later

Surgery

— Non-viable gut resected (usually very difficult to define extent of viable bowel)
— Measure accurately the length and type of gut remaining and record full details with diagram
— Free ends of gut to enterostomies rather than anastomoses
— Continuity restored later

Complications

— Stricture is common with or without surgery
— Lactose intolerance may occur (see p. 63)
— Problems associated with short gut (see p. 168)

2 THE ACUTE ABDOMEN AND OTHER SURGICAL PROBLEMS

THE ACUTE ABDOMEN

— Assessment particularly difficult in young children
— Parent history often limited
— Signs often minimal
— 90% of children with acute abdominal pain do not require emergency surgery
— See also recurrent abdominal pain (pp. 101–106)

Aetiology

— Common causes of acute abdomen in adults feature rarely in children
  • e.g. peptic ulcer, biliary tract disease, gynaecological conditions
— Less common causes in Table 2.1 have been included because they need to be recognised for appropriate management

Clinical features

History

— May be very limited in infants
— Time of onset and severity of pain
— Site, radiation and character in older children
— Associated symptoms
  • Vomiting of gastric contents or bile stained fluid
  • Dysphagia
  • Change in bowel habit
  • Haematuria, dysuria

Physical examination

— Warm environment
— Unhurried and relaxed
— General physical state especially skin and respiratory tract
— Thin abdominal wall enables more information to be obtained than in adults, e.g. general or localised distension, peristalsis
— General palpation on same principles as in adults

Table 2.1 Important causes of the acute abdomen in childhood

Common

Mesenteric lymphadenitis
Appendicitis
Trauma
Pyelonephritis
Henoch–Schönlein syndrome
Pneumonia
Acute intestinal obstruction (intussusception, incarcerated hernia, volvulus)
Gastroenteritis
Sickle cell crisis
Diabetic ketosis
Renal colic

Less common

Peptic ulcer disease (NB Meckel's)
Poison (lead, iron, corrosives)
Inflammatory bowel disease
Pancreatitis
Rheumatic fever
Torsion of ovarian cyst
Mittelschmerz
Porphyria
Neoplasia

— Inspection of hernial orifices
— Auscultation of abdomen
— Rectal examination by surgeon, if performed

Investigation

— Chest X-ray
— Erect and supine abdominal X-ray
— Full blood count, electrolytes and urea
— Blood culture

Management

— Exclude non-surgical remedial causes (e.g. pneumonia, urinary tract infection, acute follicular tonsillitis)
— Exclusion of real emergencies (e.g. ruptured spleen, volvulus, ruptured appendix)
— A short period (4–24 h) of observation before surgery

Mesenteric lymphadenitis

— Common condition, mimicking acute appendicitis
— Rare under 3 years and in adults
— Often associated with symptoms and signs of viraemia
— Pain often intermittent, periumbilical or in right iliac fossa
— Poorly localised tenderness and guarding
— Often associated with nausea, anorexia, vomiting and diarrhoea, pharyngotonsillitis

— If laparotomy: enlarged fleshy nodes
— May coexist with acute appendicitis
— Consider appendicectomy even if 'lilywhite'

Acute appendicitis

— Commonest abdominal emergency
— Diagnosis easily missed at extremes of age and hence high mortality in infancy

Classical clinical features

NB Many may be absent especially in infants
— Low grade fever and leucocytosis
— Anorexia and/or vomiting
— Right iliac fossa and/or central abdominal pain
— Change in bowel habit, usually constipation
— Guarding in right iliac fossa
— Rebound tenderness
— Tender mass on rectal examination

Management

— A few hours' observation without treatment often helps diagnosis
— Exclude peritonitis or appendix abscess clinically (see below)
— Proceed to surgery

Complications

Peritonitis

— Generalised tenderness and guarding
— Severe systemic illness (unless on steroids or immunosuppressives)
— Absence of bowel sounds
— Correct fluid and electrolyte balance
— Begin broad spectrum, antibacterial therapy including metronidazole
— Proceed to surgery

Appendix abscess

— Signs of localised peritonitis
  • Palpable mass in right iliac fossa
  • Subacute presentation
— History 24–48 h, proceed to surgery
— History longer than 48 h, and condition of patient not deteriorating
  • Conservative management
  • Intravenous fluids and antibiotics as in peritonitis
  • 'Interval' appendicectomy after 2–3 months

Postoperative abscess

— Local or wound
— Left iliac fossa
— Pelvic

— Subdiaphragmatic
— Surgical drainage and appropriate antibiotics including metronidazole

Intussusception

Incidence
— 1–2/1000 live births
— Commonest presentation at 3 months to 2 years

Aetiology
— Invagination of one segment of bowel into another
— Commonest is of terminal ileum into caecum
— Sometimes caused by polyp, Meckel's diverticulum or reduplication cyst

Features
— Brief recurring attacks of abdominal pain
  • Legs drawn up, pallor, sweating, tachycardia
— Vomiting becomes bile stained
— Blood and mucus passed per rectum
  • 'Red-currant jelly stools' (75% of cases)
— Abdominal distension
— Sausage-shaped mass
  • Often curved and concave to the umbilicus
  • Tender
  • Palpation may trigger colicky pain
— Rectal examination
  • 'Red-current jelly stools'
  • Occasionally convex mass (the head of intussusceptum)

Diagnosis
— Clinical features as above
  NB Only a few of these may be present
— Straight abdominal X-ray
  • Features of obstruction
  • Radio-opaque mass with crescentic shadow
  • May be normal
— Ultrasound
  • Mass with characteristic echoes of multiple concentric layers of intestine
— Barium enema
  • Obstruction of upward flow by convex intussusceptum

Management
Barium reduction
— Used in most cases if there is no indication for surgery (see below)
— Light sedation only (e.g. Diazepam)
— Barium introduced into rectum by Foley catheter attached to a reservoir

- Catheter is inserted, bag inflated, buttocks strapped together and catheter pulled down to anus
- Reservoir raised slowly 0.5 to 1 m above the patient with intermittent screening of abdomen
- If no evidence of reduction after 10 minutes, procedure should be abandoned

Surgery
— Indications
  - Delayed diagnosis (>24 h)
  - Shocked patient
  - Evidence of peritonitis
  - Failure of barium reduction
— Technique
  - Irreducible or non-viable intestine resected
  - End to end anastomosis
  - If reduced check for Meckel's diverticulum, polyp or reduplication
  - Consider appendicectomy

Prognosis
— Mortality 1%; nearly all late diagnosis or surgery
— Recurrence rate about 5%

Volvulus

— See p. 10

Incarcerated hernia

— Indirect inguinal by far the commonest
— Male to female ratio 10:1
— May occur in infancy so that early elective herniotomy is recommended
— Internal herniae are indistinguishable clinically from volvulus, etc.

Henoch–Schönlein syndrome

— Simulates an acute 'surgical' abdomen
— Other features suggest diagnosis
  NB But may not appear until several days after presentation with acute abdomen
— Characteristic distribution of purpuric rash
  - Commonly over extensor surfaces of limbs
— Arthropathy
— Haematuria
— Angio-oedema
— Stools usually positive for occult blood

— Melaena may occur
— Intussusception may complicate the disease
— Recurrence of episode common

Meckel's diverticulitis

— Mimics acute appendicitis
— Uncommon because of wide neck of appendage

OTHER SURGICAL PROBLEMS

Caustic oesophagitis

— Ingestion of strong alkali or acid
— Do not induce vomiting or attempt gastric lavage
— Emergency endoscopy
— Placement of large bore silastic tube as an oesophageal splint during recovery
— Empty stomach and neutralise contents
— Steroids to reduce scarring
  • Prednisolone (2 mg/kg/day for three weeks)
— Oesophagoscopy and barium swallow usually at 7–10 days
— Regular oesophagoscopy and dilatation
— Oesophageal replacement may be required

Swallowed foreign bodies

— Objects which reach the stomach are usually eventually passed per rectum
— Visualisation by X-ray is attempted
— Indications for surgery
  • Abdominal pain or tenderness
  • Failure of progression of sharp objects

Bezoars

— Accumulation of foreign material in the stomach
  • Trichobezoars – hair from self or woollen furnishings, toys, etc.
  • Phytobezoar – vegetable matter
  • Lactobezoar – milk
  • Polybezoar – mixed
— Presentation
  • Abdominal pain
  • Vomiting

- Mobile gastric mass
— Diagnosis
  - Filling defect on contrast studies
  - Endoscopy
— Management
  - Surgical except for lactobezoars which may be broken up endoscopically
  - Peritoneal soiling at operation is a significant hazard

Rectal prolapse

Incidence

— Common in infancy until growth results in an angulation at the anorectal junction
— Common in chronic diarrhoea, for example cystic fibrosis

Clinical features

— Usually symptomless prolapse noted by parent
— May be associated with mucus or blood in stool
— Reproduced by defecation in squatting position
— Rectal examination may reveal a polyp

Management

— Ensure that disorder is not intussusception
— Conservative management
  - Stool softening agents and bran
  - Strapping of buttocks together between bowel actions
— Operation may be necessary
  - In children with neurological cause, e.g. spina bifida, paraplegia
  - In incarcerated procidentia (rare)
— Exclusion of cystic fibrosis probably not warranted unless other clinical features support diagnosis

3 ACUTE DIARRHOEA AND VOMITING – GASTROENTERITIS

Gastroenteritis

- An inappropriate term for a recognised syndrome of an acute infectious disease characterised by watery diarrhoea and vomiting
- Food poisoning by toxins is not included in the term though management of dehydration is identical

Epidemiology

In industrialised societies

- Remains a significant cause of morbidity and hospital admission
- Severe metabolic disturbance is much commoner in infants, especially under 6 months of age
- Fatalities are now unusual

In developing countries

- A major continuing problem of child health
- Accounts for up to 50% of childhood morbidity and mortality
- Occurs against a background of chronic diarrhoea and malnutrition
- Reduction in mortality from this cause is a major programme for WHO for the 1990s

Predisposing factors

- Low socioeconomic status
  - Overcrowding
  - Poor sanitation
  - Non-mains supply of drinking water
- Bottle-feeding (see Table 3.1)

Table 3.1 Mechanisms by which breast milk protects against gastroenteritis

Sterile
IgA content
Lactoferrin – conjugates iron essential for growth of *E. coli*
Antiviral factors
Production of bifido bacterial colonic flora – suppresses non-lactose fermenting enteropathogens, e.g. *Shigella, Salmonella*

   — Poor nutrition predisposes to prolonged symptoms (differences also apparent in industrialised societies)
   — Abnormalities of the gastrointestinal tract
      • Low gastric acidity (e.g. due to malnutrition)
      • Reduced bowel motility (e.g. due to opiate ingestion)
      • Abnormal bowel flora (e.g. due to antibiotics)

Infecting agents

Recent advances in knowledge of pathogens
   — See Table 3.2
   — Rotavirus commonest single pathogen in infants
      • Seasonal peaks in incidence (UK – December to February)
      • Often preceding respiratory illness
      • Severe illness mostly in children under 2 years
      • Often found in neonates without symptoms
   — *Campylobacter jejuni* commonest invasive pathogen
      • Classically pain and bloody diarrhoea
      • May be fairly severe prostrating illness
      • Often prolonged (10–14 days) course
      • Erythromycin indicated for severe, prolonged illness
   — Recognition of *Giardia lamblia* as an acute diarrhoea pathogen

Table 3.2 Intestinal pathogens thought to cause acute diarrhoea and/or vomiting

Viruses
  Rotavirus
  Parvovirus (Norwalk, Hawaii, Bristol, etc.)
  Small round virus (Astro, Calici)
  Corona like virus
  Adenovirus

Bacteria
  Campylobacter jejuni (I)
  Shigellae (I)
  Salmonella (I)
  Escherichia coli ($\pm$ I)
  Yersinia enterocolitica (I)
  Vibrio cholerae
  Vibrio parahaemolyticus
  Clostridium perfringens and *difficile*
  Staphlococci
  Bacillus cereus

Parasites
  Entamoeba histolytica
  Giardia lamblia
  Cryptosporidium

I, 'Invasive' organism which may cause dysenteric stools.

— Identification of *Cryptosporidium* as a pathogen in humans
  • Of major importance in immunodeficient patients
  • No useful drug available
— Elucidation of mechanisms of bacterial diarrhoea
  • Pathophysiology of enterotoxin induced secretion
  • Demonstration of adherence factors related to *Escherichia coli*
  • Discovery of enterohaemorrhagic *E. coli* as the cause of diarrhoea associated (D+) haemolytic uraemic syndrome

Diagnosis of specific pathogen
— Important for consideration of antibiotic therapy
— Clinical features may give useful clues
  • Prodromal illness suggests viral agent
  • Abdominal pain, blood and mucus in stools suggests invasive organism
  • Rotavirus stools said to have characteristic smell identifiable by experienced staff
  • Cryptosporidial stools often watery brown, offensive
  • Enterohaemorrhagic *E. coli* can produce stools resembling pure blood
— Investigation is indicated in
  • Immunodeficient patients
  • Severely ill children
  • Outbreaks, even if small numbers of patients
  • History of foreign travel
  • Bloody diarrhoea
  • With persistent symptoms (>10 days)
  NB Best within 24–48 h of onset of symptoms for higher diagnosis rate
— Direct microscopy of stool
  • Red cells and/or pus cells suggests invasive pathogen
  • *Giardia lamblia*, *Entamoebae* or *Cryptosporidium*
  • *Campylobacter jejuni* (Gram-negative vibrios)
— EM of stool filtrate
— Culture of stool by appropriate techniques for specific pathogens
— ELISA test for rotavirus or adenovirus

Clinical features

— Significant prodromal illness uncommon except in viral episodes
— Vomiting often precedes diarrhoea by up to 48 h
— Severity of diarrhoea often underestimated by:
  • Pooling of secretions in gut
  • Liquid stool mistaken for urine in napkins
— Fever more frequent with invasive organisms but of no diagnostic value

- Should be assessed in its own right (see Differential diagnosis)
- May result in febrile convulsions
— Abdominal pain may persist (see *Campylobacter* above)

Dehydration
— Accurate, immediate assessment critical to good management
— Signs easily missed by the layman or inexperienced attendant
— Signs less apparent in hypernatraemia (see Table 3.3) and obesity
— Difficult to estimate in severe malnutrition

Table 3.3 Classical signs of normonatraemic* dehydration

Body weight loss (%)	Severity	Clinical state	Signs
<5	Mild	Not unwell	Dry mucous membranes: thirst
5–10	Moderate	Apathetic Unwell	Sunken eyes, sunken fontanelle in infants; reduced tissue elasticity, tachypnoea, oliguria
10–15	Severe	Shocked	Peripheral circulatory failure Hypotension, peripheral vasoconstriction, tachycardia
>15	Critical	Moribund	Severely shocked

* Hyponatraemia – mucous membranes tend to remain wet and excessive salivation may occur. Hypernatraemia – tissue elasticity and peripheral circulation is maintained until late. Cerebral irritation occurs early. Under-estimation of degree of dehydration is likely.

Hypernatraemia
— Less common in recent years in UK
- Humanised milks
- More emphasis on accurate making of feeds
- Possible change in epidemiology with young infants affected less
- See below for management

Differential diagnosis (see Table 3.4)
— Consider systemic infection especially meningitis
— Consider surgical emergencies particularly if
- Subacute presentation
- Vomiting
- Bile stained vomiting
- Gross abdominal distention/tenderness
- Blood in stool
- Redness or oedema of abdominal wall
— Test urine or blood for sugar

Table 3.4 Differential diagnosis of acute diarrhoea and/or vomiting

Gastroenteritis

Food poisoning

Systemic infections
  Septicaemia
  Meningitis
  Urinary tract infections
  Respiratory tract infections

Surgical conditions
  Appendicitis
  Intussusception
  Hirschsprung's disease
  Pyloric stenosis

Metabolic conditions
  Diabetic precoma
  Congenital adrenal insufficiency
  Haemolytic uraemic syndrome

Miscellaneous
  Coeliac disease
  Chronic inflammatory bowel disease
  Immune deficiency states
  Selective inborn errors of absorption
  Cow's milk protein intolerance
  Enterocolitis
  Poisoning

Investigation

Weight
  — Importance of regular weighing is usually underestimated
    • Allows objective assessment of history in outpatients during treatment
    • Allows objective measure of success in rehydration
    • Alerts clinician to underlying disorder if rehydrated weight is lower than expected for age

Biochemistry
  — Mild dehydration – none necessary
  — Moderate/severe dehydration
    • Plasma electrolytes, creatinine and glucose
    • Blood gas if clinically acidotic or total bicarbonate <10 mmol/l
  — Critical
    • Do not delay treatment if venepuncture difficult
    • Above investigation including blood gas after initial resuscitation

Microbiology
  — Stools – see above. Diagnosis of specific pathogen
  — Urine
  — Blood culture if septicaemic illness or critical condition
  — CSF examination if in doubt

Management

Oral rehydration therapy

- Effective in >90% moderately dehydrated patients when used
- Preferred in hypernatraemic dehydration
- Depends on appropriate concentrations of Na^+ and carbohydrate for its effect
- A variety of solutions are now available in the UK (Table 3.5)
- Home-made solutions can be ineffective or dangerous and are largely superseded
- Sucrose is as effective as glucose and often cheaper and more readily available
- Rice gruel and other cereal based formulae are now undergoing successful trials in developing countries
- Vomiting is not usually a contraindication
  - Often transient
  - Small frequent feed of oral rehydration fluid retained
  - Administration by continuous nasogastric infusion sometimes helpful

Table 3.5 Solutions recommended for treatment of acute diarrhoea and vomiting

	Composition (mmol/l)					
	Sodium	Potassium	Bicarbonate	Citrate	Chloride	Glucose
Dioralyte (Rorer)	60	20	–	10	60	90
Electrolade (Nicholas)	50	20	30	–	40	111
Glucose electrolyte mixture (Martindale)	35	20	18	–	37	200
Oral rehydration solution (WHO/UNICEF)	90	20	–	10	90	111

Intravenous rehydration therapy

- Indicated for patients with
  - Critical (severe) dehydration (>10% dehydrated)
  - Coma
  - ? Acute abdomen
  - Ileus
- Often required if stool output excessive (>10 ml/kg/24 h) but administration or oral rehydration solution by continuous nasogastric infusion may suffice

Treatment protocol

- See Figure 3.1

Rehydration

- Severe dehydration
  NB In the critically dehydrated infant volume expansion is an emergency
  - Treat in the admitting room/accident department of the hospital where the child is first seen

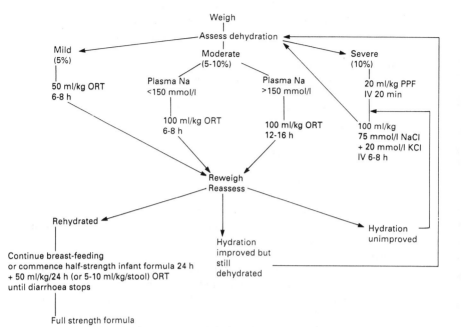

Figure 3.1 Management of acute diarrhoeal dehydration. ORT, oral rehydration therapy with Paedialyte R, Electrolade or WHO/UNICEF solutions. PPF, purified protein fraction, albumin, plasma, Haemaccel or 150 mmol/l NaCl. KCl added when urine output established

- Give IV 150 mM NaCl, plasma, albumin, purified protein fraction (PPF), Haemaccel (Hoechst/Albert) (20 ml/kg over 20 minutes)
- 150 mM NaCl as effective as colloid
— 100 ml/kg 75 mmol/l NaCl is given over 4–6 h, adding 20 mmol/l KCl if urine output established
- Further rehydration can be administered by the oral route
— Moderate dehydration is treated by administration of 100 ml/kg of oral rehydration solution over 6–8 h
— Dioralyte (Rorer), Electrolade (Nicholas), or WHO/UNICEF are preferred
- The higher Na^+ content in these solutions results in more efficient Na^+ absorption and hence correction of dehydration
— The higher carbohydrate content of Rehidrat (Searle) predisposes to hypernatraemia
— Mild dehydration is treated by administration of 50 ml/kg of oral rehydration solution over 6–8 h

NB If hypernatraemic dehydration is present (serum $Na^+ >$ 150 mmol/l)
- Use same volumes of oral rehydration solutions administered over 12–16 h, rather than 6–8 h

— If a solution of lower Na^+ concentration (<35 mmol/l) is used then 200 ml/kg should be administered over 24 h (150 mmol/kg in hypernatraemic dehydration)

Monitoring of treatment
  — Dehydrated patients require monitoring of
    • BP
    • Number and consistency of stools
    • Number and size of vomitus
    • Oral intake
    • Urine output
    • Weight change
  — Reassess after rehydration phase
  — If no improvement, rehydrate intravenously
  — If improved but signs of dehydration still present give further rehydration solution according to the mild dehydration regimen (see above)

Maintenance of fluid balance
  — 50–100 ml/kg/24 (or 5–10 ml/kg/stool) of oral rehydration solution is administered until the stools have returned to normal
    • All the solutions in Table 3.5 are suitable as maintenance fluids
  — Normal fluid requirement is provided by dietary intake (see below Nutrition)
  — If dehydration recurs, further oral rehydration solution is administered according to the regimen for rehydration (see below)

Nutrition
  — Breast-fed infants continue to receive breast milk throughout treatment
  — After rehydration infants receiving infant formulae are offered their accustomed feed at one-half strength for 24 h then full strength formula
  — Children on a mixed diet are offered their usual foods

Acute complications

Oliguria (<1 ml/kg/h)
  — Indicates either continuing dehydration or acute renal failure
  — Distinguish by
    • Urine:plasma creatinine ratio >1.1
    • Urine:plasma urea ratio >7
  — Very high concentration of plasma urea (>50 mmol/l) compatible with simple dehydration
  — If oliguric after 8 h treatment give frusemide 1 mg/kg IV
  — If oliguria persists after frusemide and urine quality is inadequate

- Urine:plasma creatinine ratio <1.1 or urine:plasma urea ratio >7
- Start renal failure regimen
  - Fluid 80 ml/kg/24 h for first day then 30–40 ml/kg/24 h + volume of previous 24 h urine output
  - No added K^+ in first 24 h
  - Acute renal failure necessitates fluid restriction
— Haematuria or palpable renal mass suggest renal vein thrombosis
  - Confirm by ultrasound and/or intravenous urography
— Persistence of polyuric phase of recovery with inappropriate sodium loss suggests permanent renal damage
  - Confirm by intravenous urography (medullary necrosis)
  - Complete functional recovery is the rule

NB Oliguria occurs in acute renal failure complicating D+ haemolytic uraemic syndrome

Hypernatraemia
— See above (Rehydration) and below (Convulsions)

Hyperkalaemia
— Complication of acute renal failure
— Serum K^+ 7.5 mmol/l in the presence of ECG changes requires emergency treatment
  - IV calcium gluconate (0.5 ml/kg of 10% solution) given over several minutes with ECG control
  - Correction of acidosis with sodium bicarbonate lowers plasma K^+ but will exacerbate any pre-existing Na^+ overload

Convulsions
— Febrile or indicating fluid/electrolyte imbalance
  NB Exclude meningitis
— In hypernatraemic dehydration fits due to hypernatraemia are more damaging than those due to rapid rehydration
— Correction of hypocalcaemia rarely stops convulsions
— Prophylaxis
  - Phenobarbitone in severe hypernatraemia
— Treatment
  - Diazepam (IV) and
  - Phenobarbitone thereafter 10 mg/kg/24 h
  - Consider dexamethasone in established cerebral oedema

Hypokalaemia
— Presents as hypotension or bradycardia during rehydration
— ECG shows flattened T waves, U waves and prolonged QT interval
— Malnourished children at particular risk
— IV correction requires ECG control
  - IV fluids should not contain more than 80 mmol/l K^+
  - Hyperkalaemia causes tall peaked T waves, flattened P waves and widening of the QRS complex

Pulmonary oedema
- — Due to simple overload
- — Commoner with acidosis
- — Treatment
  - • IV frusemide
  - • Positive pressure ventilation

Hyperglycaemia
- — Commonly accompanies hypernatraemia
- — Patients show extreme insulin sensitivity
- — Self-correcting as serum Na^+ is reduced

Further management

Antidiarrhoeal agents
- NB Not indicated in management of acute diarrhoea in an infant
- — Traditional use of absorbent powders and opiates
- — Superseded by opiate analogues such as loperamide
  - • Contraindications include liver disease
- — Do not use diphenoxylate
  - • Overdosage by both doctor and parent (occasionally fatal) has been described
- — Socially desirable effects in older children and adults

Antibiotics
- — Widely prescribed but have a very limited role (see Table 3.6)
  - • Most infections are viral
  - • Most bacterial diarrhoea self-limiting
  - • Not indicated in enterohaemorrhagic *E. coli* diarrhoea
- — Use has been suggested to reduce crossinfection in hospitalised patients but adequate trial data are lacking
- — Definite indications for their use are given in Table 3.6 and Figure 3.2

Table 3.6 Indications for antimicrobial therapy in diarrhoeal disease

Severe *Shigella* infection
Systemic salmonellosis
Typhoid and paratyphoid fever
Campylobacter infection when severe or prolonged
Cholera
Yersinia enterocolitica infection
Diagnostic doubt between septicaemia and gastroenteritis
Amoebic dysentery
Giardiasis

Management in the older child (over 2 years)

- — Malnourished children managed as infants (Figure 3.1)
- — Well-nourished children managed broadly as adults (Figure 3.2)

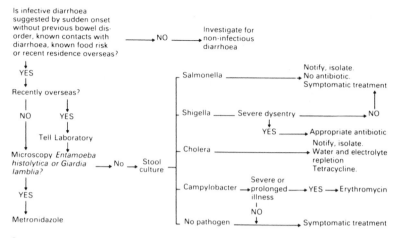

Figure 3.2 Management of gastroenteritis in the older child (after Lambert *Clin. Gastroenterol.* Sept. 1979)

Later complications

Failure of diarrhoea to resolve

— Recurrence of some diarrhoea during regrading is common (10–30%)
  • 'Going back' to clear fluids is usually unnecessary
  • Lactose intolerance sometimes occurs in this phase
— Persistent lactose intolerance (lasting more than 10 days) now uncommon
  • Lactose-free diet is indicated (see Appendix B)
— Intolerance to cow's milk protein or any oral feed may supervene, rarely
  • Commonly termed postenteritis syndrome
  • Management is by special diet and possibly intravenous nutrition

Prognosis

— Major cause of child mortality in developing and less industrialised countries
  • May account for 50% of deaths of children under 5 years
— Significant morbidity associated with:
  • Hypernatraemia – cerebral palsy and mental retardation
  • Postenteritis syndrome – prolonged malnutrition
  • Chronic renal problems after severe dehydration
  • D+ haemolytic uraemic syndrome is the commonest cause of acute renal failure in children in northern Europe

4 GASTROINTESTINAL COMPLICATIONS OF IMMUNOSUPPRESSION, CYTOTOXIC THERAPY AND AIDS

— Cytotoxic therapy and resulting bone marrow and immuno-suppression result in a number of serious gastrointestinal problems
— AIDS presents very similar problems and is becoming much more widely studied and understood
  • Associated with a greater variety of infectious agents

Septicaemia

— The commonest complication of cytotoxic therapy
— GI organisms are common pathogens
— 'Sterilisation' of the gut in patients particularly at risk (e.g. pre-bone marrow transplant) is practised in some centres
  • Carries risks of colonising unit with resistant organisms
— Often related to indwelling catheters, central lines, etc.

Oesophagitis

— Pain on swallowing in patients receiving chemotherapy may be due to
  • Fungal oesophagitis
    – Usually candidal
  • Herpetic oesophagitis
    – Usually with mouth affected also
    – Swallowing difficulty
    – Systemic treatment

Vomiting

— Associated with drug therapy
— With oesophagitis
— In paralytic ileus
— Associated with bacterial, fungal or viral infections

Prolonged infectious diarrhoea

— GI organisms which are commonly invasive may give rise to septicaemia
— GI organisms which usually result in a self-limiting diarrhoeal illness may cause prolonged severe diarrhoea and malabsorption
— e.g. *Giardia, Cryptosporidium, Salmonella, Shigella, Campylobacter, Helicobacter*, rotavirus and other viruses

Malnutrition

— Failure to thrive/malnutrition is very common
— Good nutrition is very important in successful management of the underlying disorder
— Poor intake is almost the rule in patients on chemotherapy and must be distinguished from malabsorption
— Use dietary supplements, nasogastric feeding with elemental diets or intravenous nutrition if nausea or vomiting is a problem
  • Check stools for sugars

Malabsorption

— Immunodeficiency may present as protracted diarrhoea
— Often associated with bacterial overgrowth of the small intestine
— Also possible decreased enterocyte production directly due to drug or radiation therapy or graft versus host disease
  • Subtotal villous atrophy
  • Lactose intolerance
— Manage as protracted diarrhoea (p. 41)

Acute enterocolitis

— An occasional complication with sudden dramatic deterioration
— Commonly affects ileocaecal region (Tiflitis)
Associations
— High risk situations include
  • Radiation in combination with chemotherapy
  • High dose cyclophosphamide
  • Combined regimens (e.g. those for induction of remission) or intensification phases of ALL treatments
  • CMV infection
Presentation
— Severity of symptoms may be masked by
  • Neutropenia and poor physical response
  • Immunosuppression due to steroids
— Acute bloody diarrhoea
— Acute abdominal distension

— Intestinal obstruction/ileus etc.
— Septicaemia
— Acute phase reactants often raised

Management

— Septicaemia is nearly always present
  • Broad spectrum antibiotics such as an aminoglycoside and piperacillin together with metronidazole
  • Look for *Clostridium difficile* and toxin and include vancomycin if toxin present or occasionally with culture positive only
— Frequent X-rays to detect perforation
— Regular clinical assessment e.g. 4–6 hourly
— Delay surgical intervention for 24–48 h if no perforation
— Neutrophil transfusion (rarely useful)
— Careful attention to fluid and electrolyte balance

Graft versus host disease

— Affects up to 50% of patients post bone-marrow transplant

Acute

— Skin rashes
  • Often non-specific, maculopapular
— Cholestatic liver disease
  • Initially only biochemical evidence of disturbed liver function

Fulminant

— Severe exfoliative dermatitis
— Hepatic failure
— Severe debilitating diarrhoea

Chronic

— Later onset
— Progressive sclerodermatous skin reaction
— Liver changes mimicking primary biliary cirrhosis in some patients

5 CHRONIC DIARRHOEA, INFLAMMATORY BOWEL DISEASE AND MALABSORPTION

Definitions of diarrhoea

Lay
 — Change in stool consistency towards looseness
 — Increase in stool frequency
 — Incontinence of soft faeces or liquid staining

Medical
 — Increase in stool water
 — Usually based on history and observation rather than measurement
 • But severity can usefully be measured by simple weight (e.g. double weighing of nappies with urine collected separately)

Spurious diarrhoea
 — Constipation and overflow or liquid soiling often mistaken by patient as diarrhoea
 — History confuses physician who treats for diarrhoea (see p. 108)
 — Frequent small volume stools may be confusing in infants after diarrhoea

---

CHRONIC DIARRHOEA WITHOUT FAILURE TO THRIVE

Breast-feeding
 — Many breast-fed infants have 5–8 'loose' stools daily

Toddler diarrhoea (chronic non-specific diarrhoea of infancy, irritable bowel syndrome of infancy)

Clinical features
 — Onset between 6 months and 2 years

— Commoner in boys
— Variable pattern of stool consistency and frequency
— Diarrhoea may alternate with constipation
— First stool of the day may be formed
— Exacerbated by high roughage diet, e.g. fruit, Weetabix
— Stools contain undigested vegetable lumps, e.g. peas, carrots, etc.
— Stools contain mucus
— Child remains well and thrives
— 'Disorder' tends to decrease with age
  • Rarely persists beyond 6 years

Diagnosis

— By recognition of clinical features
— Check growth velocity
— Exclude giardiasis (p. 61) and carbohydrate intolerance

Further management

— Reassurance of parents
— Acceptance of healthy child, albeit with loose stools
  • Probably delay in maturation of motility
  • Growth is normal
  • Not associated with delay in achieving continence
— If severe may extend investigation to exclude malabsorption
— If causing family distress consider using loperamide
  • May reinforce parent's suspicion of bowel disease

Sucrose intolerance

— May present with failure to thrive (see p. 73)
— Often does not present until weaning as sugar now rarely added to milk feeds
— Autosomal recessive disorder commoner than congenital lactase deficiency
— Secondary deficiency uncommon as the enzyme less liable to damage by mucosal insults but may be affected in severe protein energy malnutrition
— May present acutely in infants given sucrose-containing feeds
— May be mild due to partial deficiency of sucrase/isomaltase
— May not cause failure to thrive (unlike lactose intolerance which in infants often causes FTT)
— Exclude by testing a fresh watery stool for carbohydrate
  NB must be boiled first with HCl to hydrolyse sucrose
— If confirmed avoid sucrose in diet except in tolerated amounts
— If severe may also need to reduce starch intake
— Severity of symptoms lessen with age

CHRONIC DIARRHOEA WITH FAILURE TO THRIVE — PROTRACTED DIARRHOEA

Definition
— Passage of four or more loose stools a day for more than two weeks with associated failure to thrive

Differential diagnosis
— See Table 5.1
— Major 'idiopathic' group

Table 5.1 Differential diagnosis of protracted diarrhoea of infancy

Causes	Examples
Food protein intolerance	Coeliac disease Cow's milk protein intolerance Soy protein intolerance Other protein intolerance
Carbohydrate intolerance	Glucose/galactose malabsorption Secondary monosaccharide intolerance Sucrase/isomaltase deficiency Lactase deficiency Secondary lactose intolerance
Other selective inborn errors of absorption	Congenital chloridorrhoea Transcobalamin II deficiency Acrodermatitis enteropathica Defective Na^+/H^+ exchange
Surgical	Malrotation Hirschsprung's disease Stenosis Blind loop syndrome
Extraintestinal infections	Abscess
Intestinal infections	Enteropathogenic *E. coli* *Giardia lamblia* Dysenteric infections
Antibiotics	Pseudomembranous colitis
Pancreatic insufficiency	Cystic fibrosis Shwachman syndrome
Immunodeficiency	Severe combined immunodeficiency Hypogammaglobulinaemia Defective yeast opsonisation AIDS
Tumours	Ganglioneuroma Lymphoma Histiocytosis X
Chronic inflammatory bowel disease	Ulcerative colitis Crohn's disease
Other	Necrotising enterocolitis Addison's disease Lymphangiectasia Congenital microvillous atrophy Autoimmune enteropathy
Unknown	Familial protracted diarrhoea

History (useful pointers)

— Association of onset with introduction of cow's milk (intolerance) or cereals (coeliac disease)
— Abdominal pain, borborygmi, frothy, watery stools (carbohydrate intolerance)
— Alternating diarrhoea, vomiting and constipation (surgical causes, malrotation, Hirschsprung's, stenoses, Crohn's)
— Family history (inborn errors of absorption, immune deficiency, cystic fibrosis)
— Bloody diarrhoea (inflammatory bowel disease)

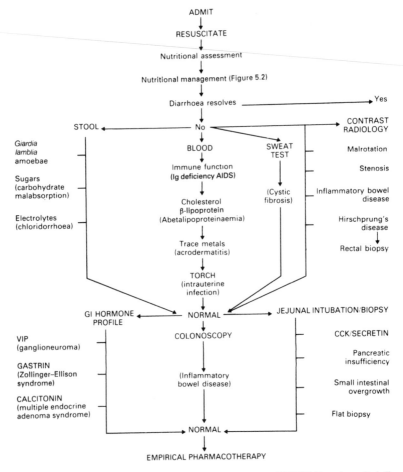

Figure 5.1 Management and investigation of protracted diarrhoea. TORCH, Toxoplasma Rubella CMV and Herpes serology

Examination

Diagnostic (rarely helpful)
- Gross abdominal distention (surgical disorders and congenital chloridorrhoea)
- Increased bowel sounds (subacute obstruction)
- Chest signs (cystic fibrosis and immunodeficiency)
- Oedema (protein losing enteropathy)

Dehydration (see Chapter 3)
- May be difficult to assess
  - Signs such as enophthalmos, poor tissue turgor present in malnutrition without dehydration
  - Look for dry mouth and poor peripheral perfusion

Nutrition
- Compare admission height, rehydrated weight, and head circumference with previous measurements
- Assess skinfold thickness on percentile chart
- Height and head circumference affected by prolonged malnutrition

Investigation
- See Figure 5.1

Management (See Figures 5.1 and 5.2)
- Resuscitation and rehydration
- Nutritional support
- Treat diagnosed disorder

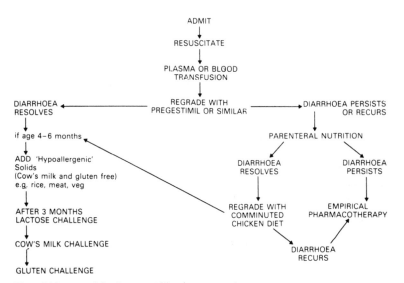

Figure 5.2 Protracted diarrhoea – nutritional management

Further treatment of protracted diarrhoea when no causative diagnosis established

— Treatment of possible 'mechanisms'
  - Trimethoprim/metronidazole for small intestinal bacterial overgrowth
  - Cholestyramine, if bile acid deconjugation demonstrated (bile salt binding resin – may exacerbate total bile salt deficiency, and fat soluble vitamin deficiency)
— Empirical therapy
  - Na cromoglycate (Nalcrom) if history suggests dietary protein intolerance
  - Prednisolone (1–2 mg/kg/day) for 10 days. If no response, steroids should be withdrawn
  - Loperamide in high dosage. May cause ileus

CONDITIONS CLASSICALLY ASSOCIATED WITH MALABSORPTION/DIARRHOEA/FTT

Coeliac disease

Prevalence

— Variable in the UK
  - Average for UK 1 in 2000
  - West Eire 1 in 300
— Falling in recent years in childhood
— Familial pattern
  - Not simple mendelian inheritance
  - 10% of first-degree relatives affected

Aetiology

— Toxic effects of cereal protein (gluten)
  - Alpha-gliadin protein
— Glutens vary in toxicity
  - Wheat > rye > barley > oats
  - Maize (corn) and rice gluten non-toxic

Pathology

— Small intestinal mucosa affected
  - Proximal intestine ≫ distal (distal not exposed to gluten)
— 'Subtotal villous atrophy'
  - Loss of villous pattern
  - Crypt hypertrophy
  - Surface columnar epithelium becomes cuboid and disrupted
  - Increased intraepithelial lymphocytes

- Plasma cell infiltrate of lamina propria
- Increased mitotic figures in crypts
— EM appearance
  - Damaged brush border
  - Increased cell loss
  - Immature cells
— Functional studies
  - Immature epithelial cells (crypt like)
  - Low lactase activity
  - Low (Na^+-K^+)-ATPase activity
  - Intestine in net secretory state
  NB Appearances are not unique for coeliac disease (see below)

Clinical features

Classical

— Growth failure after introduction of cereals (variable latent period)
  - Weight more affected than height or head circumference
— Abnormal faeces
  - Frequent, soft, pale
  NB not invariable – constipation may occur
— Anorexia – 'fussy eaters'
— Irritability
— Vomiting
— Abdominal distension
— Muscle wasting – particularly limb girdle muscles and proximal limb muscles

Other

— Anaemia
  - Iron or folate deficient or both
— Rickets or osteomalacia
  - Particularly in at-risk groups, e.g. Asians in UK
— Lactose intolerance
  - Secondary to low mucosal lactase
— Hypoalbuminaemia + oedema
  - Due to protein losing enteropathy
— Hypoprothrombinaemia
  - Due to vitamin K malabsorption

Diagnosis

'Screening' tests

— Generally of limited value
  - Both false positives and false negatives occur
  - They add to distress of hospital experience
  - Serum and red cell folate
  - Serum iron and ferritin
  - Plasma calcium, phosphate and alkaline phosphatase
  - Xylose loading test with urine or blood analysis

- Alpha-gliadin serum antibodies usually present in untreated or relapsing coeliac disease
- Differential absorption of oligosaccharides has been used as a test of mucosal absorption and permeability
  - May be useful in detecting relapse during challenges
  - Needs confirmation by biopsy
- Barium meal and follow through

Jejunal biopsy
— Definitive test (see pp. 172–177)
— Defer only in severely ill infant
— Experienced operator and laboratory essential for proper interpretation and minimal distress to patient

Differential diagnosis of villous atrophy
— Over 1 year of age a flat biopsy is virtually pathognomonic of coeliac disease

Any age
— Coeliac disease
— Severe combined immunodeficiency
— Protein energy malnutrition
— Tropical sprue
— Autoimmune enteropathy
— Antineoplastic therapy
— Protracted diarrhoea of unknown cause

Commoner under 1 year
— Cow's milk protein intolerance
— Soy protein intolerance
— Temporary gluten intolerance
— Gastroenteritis
— Giardiasis

Management
— See Figure 5.3

Initial treatment
— Presume diagnosis of coeliac disease
— Gluten-free diet
  - Expert advice of dietitian
  - Publications of Coeliac Society (PO Box 181, London NW2 2QY, UK)
— Specific therapy for any of 'less common' clinical features (see above)
  - e.g. lactose free diet, plasma/albumin infusion, etc.
— Consider steroids in very serious case (coeliac crisis)

Preschool child
— Maintain gluten-free diet
— Monitor growth and clinical features
— Educate parents and child
— Plan confirmation of diagnosis by gluten challenge

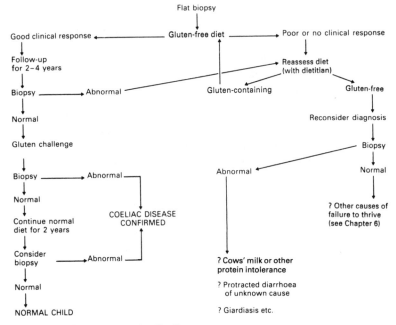

Figure 5.3 Diagnostic management of coeliac disease

Poor clinical response/relapse/diet failure
- Careful dietary check by dietitian
- Re-biopsy
- Re-evaluate diagnosis
- Re-educate parent and child if necessary

Gluten challenge
- Essential to confirm diagnosis
- Most important if initial presentation <1 year

Timing
- Delay of 2–4 years allows catch up growth
- 'Preschool' timing may solve difficulty of school meals
- Procedure can be explained to 4–6-year-olds

Prechallenge biopsy
- Must be morphologically normal to allow interpretation of post-challenge specimen

Administration of gluten
- Either gluten powder added to diet (10–15 g/day)
  - Unpleasant taste so may not be taken
  - Not a natural product
  - Parents know that it is potentially 'toxic'
- Or gluten-containing foods (15+ g/day of gluten)
  - e.g. bread 3 g/slice
  - Weetabix 5 g/biscuit

- Child may dislike gluten-containing foods
- Potential difficulties of returning to gluten-free diet

Post-challenge biopsy
— Should not be undertaken before 3–4 months post-challenge **unless** definite clinical relapse with marked symptoms confirmed in hospital
— Minor symptoms often result of patient's or parent's anxiety
— If normal morphology
  - Initial diagnosis secure (e.g. 2-year-old with flat biopsy and no other cause) then rebiopsy after 2 years on normal diet
  - Otherwise rebiopsy only if symptoms recur
— Abnormal morphology confirms diagnosis
— European Society of Gastroenterology (ESPGAN) have revised their criteria to a single biopsy showing hyperplastic villous atrophy while receiving gluten and a clinical response to gluten withdrawal
  - Loss of circulating antibodies (IgA, gliadin, antireticulin) on additional gluten withdrawal as supportive evidence

Long-term management
— Educate parents and child
  - Need for life-long diet
  - Absence of symptoms when breaking diet
— Long-term follow-up especially while growing and through pregnancy

Disorders associated with coeliac disease/gluten intolerance
— Dermatitis herpetiformis
  - Some have a gluten-sensitive enteropathy
  - Skin may also respond to gluten withdrawal
— HLA-B8 associated diseases
  - Diabetes mellitus
  - Autoimmune thyroid disease
  - Pernicious anaemia
— IgA deficiency
  - Common in coeliac disease
  - IgA deficiency may predispose
— Bowel malignancy
  - Small bowel neoplasms roughly 20 times more common in patients with coeliac disease but especially lymphoma
  - Gluten-free diet may protect

Other dietary protein intolerances with gastrointestinal manifestations

— Reactions are thought to be immunologically mediated
— Commoner in the first year of life
— Clinical manifestations are protean (see below)
— Many different proteins have been implicated

— Villous atrophy has only been demonstrated in gluten, cow's milk and soy protein intolerance
— Life-long intolerance has only been demonstrated with gluten

Clinical syndromes which may be precipitated by ingestion of cow's milk

— Acute anaphylaxis (occasional cot death?)
— Urticaria
— Eczema (often cross-sensitivity with egg albumin)
— Asthma
— Vomiting (occasionally as only manifestation)
— Watery diarrhoea (usually acute with vomiting)
— Protracted diarrhoea (= coeliac syndrome)
— Acute colitis
— Occult gastrointestinal blood loss leading to iron deficiency anaemia
— Colic
— Migraine
— Constipation

Cow's milk protein intolerance as a model

— Diagnosis and management of dietary protein intolerance may be modelled on that of cow's milk protein

Pathogenesis

— Detectable absorption of whole protein macromolecules occurs in humans
  • Increased in young infants especially preterm infants
  • Increased if infants IgA deficient
  • Results in excretion of whole protein in breast milk
— Immune 'tolerance' is usually IgA mediated
— Hypersensitivity reactions are established in some infants
  • Immediate type (usually with raised IgE and positive specific IgE as measured by Radio-Allergo Sorbent Test (RAST)
  • Delayed type
— Soluble proteins of cow's milk are most important (lactalbumin and lactoglobulins)
  • If dramatic improvement on diet do not immediately challenge (except for research!)
  • Challenge after 6–12 months but not before 12–18 months of age
  • These are present as a high proportion of the protein in most humanised formulae
— Hypersensitivity commonly occurs in atopic individuals with a family history of asthma, eczema or hay fever

Diagnosis

Diagnosis is based on clinical data

— Remission on withdrawal of cow's milk from diet
— Relapse on reintroduction
— Further remission on withdrawal

  — These criteria are sufficient for a clinical diagnosis
  — For research purposes three challenges must be followed by symptoms identical in type and time of onset

Supportive laboratory tests

  — Response to intradermal skin test with negative control
  — Positive RAST of 2+ or greater
  — Total plasma IgE raised for age
  — High eosinophil count
  — Small intestinal enteropathy 24 h after challenge

Management

Dietary trial

  — When diagnosis is suspected trial of cow's milk protein-free diet must be carefully supervised by a dietitian
  — Fully milk-fed infants may be fed on a variety of commercial preparations (Appendix B, p. 182) or possibly goat's milk (potential cross-reaction with cow's milk)
  — Mothers of breast-fed infants should be put on fully cow's milk protein-free diet
  — If these conditions are met a month's trial is nearly always sufficient

Challenge

  — Timing and interpretation
    • If no effect is apparent, return to normal diet after one month
    • No response to challenge leaves the original diagnosis in doubt
    • Positive response is indication to return to exclusion diet and repeat challenge every 6–9 months
  — Method
    • Admit and record weight
    • Carry out lactose challenge using either load method or introduction method
    • Use 'doorstep' fresh milk throughout
    • Load method
      – Skin test with cow's milk. Strong positive reaction is indication for care but not to abandon the challenge
      – Give 1 ml orally and double intake every hour to reach 32 ml at 5 hours
      – Monitor
        Stool frequency and appearance
        Temperature, pulse and respiration
      – Discharge home on increasing amounts of cow's milk diet; increase gradually to at least 250 ml/day
    • Introduction method
      – Ask parent to give 1 teaspoon milk in feed on first day, tablespoon second day then gradual increase
      – Do not abandon challenge until symptoms are definitely confirmed (except in case of suspected anaphylaxis)
    • Symptoms may take days or even weeks to reappear

Dietary relaxation
- — Diet must be strict for trial period
- — Many children do not react adversely to partially denatured protein as in cheese, yogurt or chocolate
  - • Introduce these when condition stable on diet
  - • Only one new food each 2 weeks and monitor symptoms

Prognosis
- — Clinical symptoms related to the gastrointestinal tract appear to remit spontaneously and are rare after 2 years of age
- — Long-term complications, as in coeliac patients who break their diet, have not been described

Cystic fibrosis

Genetics
- — Commonest lethal autosomal recessive condition in UK

Prevalence
- — 1 in 2000 Caucasian live births
- — 5% of population heterozygotes; suggests a selective advantage of carrier status

Pathogenesis
- — See Figure 5.4
- — Basic defect concerns electrolyte transport across cell membranes

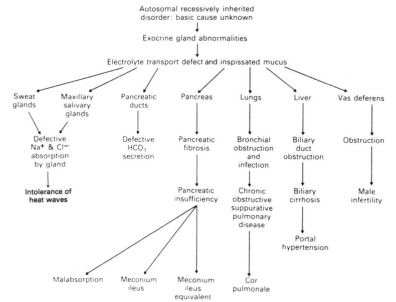

Figure 5.4 Pathogenesis of cystic fibrosis

- Chloride secretion abnormal in epithelia and exocrine glands
- Abnormal membrane protein now identified
- Informative DNA studies re heterozygotes possible in >70% (see below, Diagnosis)
— Mucus produced by exocrine glands is excessively viscid
— These glands become atrophied, secondary to duct obstruction
— Lungs become infected and develop bronchiectasis

Presenting symptoms
 — See Table 5.2

Table 5.2 Presenting features of cystic fibrosis

	Respiratory	*Gastrointestinal*	*Other*
Neonatal	Pneumonia	Meconium ileus Prolonged jaundice	Positive family history Positive screening test (See text)
Infancy and early childhood	Paroxysmal cough with vomiting Wheezing Recurrent pneumonia	Steatorrhoea Failure to thrive Polyphagia	Heat exhaustion
Later childhood	Purulent sputum Bronchiectasis Exertional dyspnoea Cor pulmonale Haemoptysis Chronic sinusitis Nasal polypi	Meconium ileus equivalent Portal hypertension Hypersplenism	Diabetes mellitus

Respiratory features
 — Recurrent chest infections
 — Productive cough frequently with sputum
 — Frequent isolation of Staphylococci or Pseudomonas in sputum
 — Overexpanded chest with moderate airways obstruction
 — Adventitious sounds are common
 — Chest X-ray shows characteristic features
   - Ring, blob and tramline shadows
   - Unlike bronchiectasis from other causes changes affect all areas of the lung fields
   - Clubbing and cyanosis may be present in older children

Gastrointestinal features
 — Meconium ileus or equivalent (see p. 11)
 — Failure to thrive associated with a ravenous appetite
 — Large, pale, exceptionally foul smelling, greasy stools
 — Deficiency of fat soluble vitamins A, D, E or K
 — Rectal prolapse (probably due to malnutrition)

Growth failure
 — Poor growth undoubtedly contributes to deterioration in lung function

— If sufficient oral intake to maintain growth impossible consider
  • Overnight tube feeding via oral, nasal or gastrostomy tube
  • IV feeding
— Good nutrition essential pretransplant

Diagnosis in children

Sweat test

  • At present the most reliable routine test
  • False negative and false positive results still occur in good centres
  • Test must be done by experienced clinical and laboratory personnel
  • Duplicate tests (one on each arm) should always be done on at least one occasion. Poor duplication suggests need for repeat test
  • Unexpected results should be interpreted in the light of clinical data and repeated
— Method
  • Prepare approximately $12\,cm^2$ blotting paper weighed inside a dry air-tight container
  • Use properly designed iontophoresis apparatus
  • Soak tissues or gauze over anode in 1% pilocarpine
  NB Burns are caused by release of acid at anode not by electric current or voltage, therefore use thick layer of padding in anode
  • Dry large area of skin very carefully
  • Apply weighted blotting paper, handling only with forceps
  • Cover with a piece of polythene overlapping by 0.5 to 1 cm only and seal with waterproof tape such as 'Sleek'
  • Leave for 30 minutes with limb wrapped in loose crepe bandage then remove plaster and lift paper with forceps to its weighing container
  • Laboratory will weigh and analyse
— Interpretation
  • At least 100 mg of sweat is required for any meaningful result
— First sweat often contains higher Na^+ than later sweat
— Larger volume also decreases importance of evaporative losses
  • Clearly positive results are in 80–120 mmol/l range
  • Borderline results are in 50–80 mmol/l range
— False positive results
  • Preterm infants or infants <3 days of age may have high results, usually in borderline range
  • Children after puberty and adults have very variable results often in cystic range
  • In severe malnutrition high values may be obtained
  • Other causes of high results usually have other suggestive clinical features and include
    – Adrenal insufficiency
    – Renal diabetes insipidus

         – Von Gierke's disease (Type 1 glycogen storage disease)
         – Fucosidosis
    — Other routine diagnostic tests
       • Ion (chloride) sensitive electrodes used on
         – Salivary secretions
         – The skin
       • Sweat osmolality

Screening tests
    — Stool trypsin – <1/80 suggests cystic fibrosis but is an unreliable test giving false positives and negatives
    — Stool chymotrypsin most reliable
    — Meconium albumin concentration using BM Meconium test
       • Unreliable though false positive rate said to be low with an experienced user
    — Plasma immunoreactive trypsin using blood collected on blotting paper (Guthrie card) raised in neonatal period

Diagnosis in equivocal cases, adults or children after puberty
    — Pancreatic function test (see p. 172)
       • Volume is decreased
       • HCO_3^- amount and concentration is decreased
       • Enzyme activities amount and concentration are decreased in about 85% of patients
    — DNA typing
       • Very useful if other family members available
       • Some value even with patient only specimen
       • Blood (or tissue) needed from an index case and both parents ideally

Management of gastrointestinal features
Malabsorption
    — High energy, high protein, normal fat diet
    — Medium chain triglyceride (MCT) may be used to replace some of the fat
    — Pancreatic enzyme supplements given in quantity that is sufficient to render stools virtually normal
       • Newer preparations such as Creon or Pancrease 2–8 g before meals allow free fat diet and a higher energy intake
       • Or Pancrex V Forte 0.5 g per feed in infancy increasing to 2–8 g with meals in children
       • Too much pancreatic supplement results in tenesmus and perineal excoriation especially in infants
    — Problem of gastric denaturation helped by
       • Newer preparation (e.g. Creon, Pancrease)
       • H_2 antagonist therapy (e.g. cimetidine)
    — Polyvitamin supplements and vitamin E 50–100 mg/day
Meconium ileus equivalent
    — Acute: As for meconium ileus – medically and if necessary surgically (p. 11)

- Gastrografin orally on 2 consecutive days
  - <25 kg 50 ml
  - 25–60 kg 100 ml
  - >60 kg 150 ml
— Chronic: Presents with non-specific abdominal pain, faeces palpable per abdomen
  - Treat with acetyl cysteine orally
  - Increase pancreatic supplement

Respiratory management
— Physiotherapy is mainstay of treatment
  - Prophylactic physiotherapy as soon as diagnosis is suspected
  - Home therapy: postural drainage and percussion
  - Intensive inpatient physiotherapy during acute infective exacerbations
  - Self-therapy with 'huffing', especially in older patients
  - Provision of foam wedge or tipping frame and/or trampoline may be very beneficial
— Antibiotics
  - Most recommend continuous antistaphylococcal antibiotic (e.g. flucloxacillin) for first year of life
  - Acute: infective exacerbations treated with 2-week course IV broad spectrum antibiotics
    - e.g. gentamicin and flucloxacillin or piperacillin
    - Plus nebulised antibiotics, e.g. gentamicin, Colomycin
  - Also used for subacute respiratory symptoms with growth failure
  - Antibiotics used freely for less severe respiratory symptoms
  - Indications for prophylactic antibiotics not defined
    - But patients with severe pulmonary involvement will be receiving virtually continuous antibiotics
  - Nebulised antibiotics used in most centres especially for patients with *Pseudomonas* colonisation
  - Dispute exists about relative benefits of continuous antibiotics
    - ? Reduced lung damage with less infection
    - Increased likelihood of early *Pseudomonas* colonisation
— Inhalation
  - Bronchodilators
  - Steroids (beclomethasone): if superimposed allergic bronchospasm
  - Na cromoglycate (Intal)
  - Mucolytics (acetyl cysteine)
— Steroids
  - Single studies suggest general improvements
    - But short term and risk of complications and increased infection

- Avoid oral steroids if possible
  - Especially if being considered for transplant
- Are used for allergic aspergillosis
— Pneumothorax
  - Manage as conservatively as possible
— Ventilation
  - Avoid if at all possible

Heart and lung transplantation
— Contraindications – avoid if possible
  - Malnutrition (can be corrected pre-operation)
  - Pleurectomy or other surgical therapy of pneumothoraces
  - Steroid therapy
— Preparation
  - Attention to nutrition
  - Aim to reduce infection by treatment of *Pseudomonas* including sinuses and upper tract

General management
— NaCl supplements in hot weather
  NB Sick infants with cystic fibrosis may present with pseudo-Barrter syndrome
  - Severe metabolic alkalosis, hypokalaemia and hyponatraemia
— Counselling
  - Stresses arise from
    - Difficulties in dilemma of how much knowledge/discussion and when
    - Declining pulmonary function
    - Failure of career, marriage, child-bearing
    - Arduous treatment programmes
    - Transplantation risk/benefit equations
— Develop close supportive relationship with paediatrician, physiotherapist, dietician, specialist nurse and social worker

Prognosis
— About 50% now live beyond the age of 20 without transplantation
— Early transplant mortality <20%
  - Long-term outlook uncertain but good quality short-term survival likely

Shwachman syndrome

— Autosomal recessive inheritance
— Much less common than cystic fibrosis

Features
— See Table 5.3

Table 5.3 Features of Shwachman syndrome

Exocrine pancreatic insufficiency (100%)

Haematological abnormalities
  Abnormal neutrophil motility (85%)
  Neutropenia (intermittent) (95%)
  Thrombocytopenia (70%)
  Raised HbF (40%)
  Anaemia (50%)
  Lymphoproliferative and myeloproliferative disorders

Growth retardation (95%)

Skeletal abnormalities
  Metaphyseal dysplasia (60%)
  Abnormal ribs
  Delayed bone age (95%)
  Tubulation of long bones (30%)
  Clinodactyly (50%)

Recurrent infections (100%)
  Variable immunoglobulin deficiency
  Impaired neutrophil motility

Hepatosplenomegaly (60%)
  Raised transaminases (80%)

Ichthyosis (80%)

Neonatal problems (80%)
  Poor feeding
  Respiratory distress

Developmental delay (90%)
  Hypotonia (20%)

Dental abnormalities
  Caries (40%)
  Dysplasia (15%)

Occasional abnormalities
  Renal tubular dysfunction
  Diabetes mellitus
  Hypertelorism
  Retinitis pigmentosa
  Endocardial fibrosis
  Hirschsprung's disease

Diagnosis

— Coincidence of clinical features with abnormal pancreatic function

NB Volume and bicarbonate output in response to secretin is normal; compare cystic fibrosis

Management

— Pancreatic enzyme supplements as in cystic fibrosis (do not improve growth)
— Vitamin supplements
— Antibiotics for acute infections
— Occasional blood transfusion may be needed (e.g. prior to surgery)

Prognosis

— Significant mortality associated with infection and malignancy
— Clinical severity quite variable
— Usually better prognosis than cystic fibrosis
— Many have variable degrees of retardation

Pancreatitis

Aetiology

Acute

— Trauma
  NB Non-accidental injury
— Viruses, particularly mumps
— Bacteria, e.g. mycoplasma
— Parasites, e.g. malaria
— Drugs (check thoroughly)
— Pancreatic duct obstruction
— Acute haemorrhagic pancreatitis
— Vasculitis, e.g. SLE, Henoch–Schönlein
— Following organ transplantation
— Inflammatory bowel disease
— Recovering malnutrition
— Idiopathic

Chronic (often calcific)

— Familial – autosomal dominant – onset in 2nd decade
— Hyperlipidaemia
— Hyperparathyroidism
— Following organ transplantation
— Autoimmune
— Lipodystrophy
— Idiopathic

Diagnosis

Acute

— Plasma amylase grossly raised
— Acute abdomen with peritonism

Chronic

— Recurrent abdominal pain
— Pancreatic calcification on straight X-ray or ultrasound
— Abnormal pancreatic function tests

Management

Acute

— Treat shock with plasma and blood transfusions
— Analgaesia
— Nasogastric aspiration
— IV calcium supplements as required

Chronic
— Pancreatic supplements
— Low fat diet

Gastrointestinal parasites causing protracted diarrhoea

Diagnosis
— By demonstration of eggs, in larval or adult forms in freshly prepared faecal material

Strongyloides **(roundworm)**

Area
— Tropics and subtropics

Life cycle
— Larvae penetrate skin to lungs to bronchi to gut
— Adults mature in small intestines – eggs mature to larvae in same host or to new human host via faeces or autoinfect (hence perpetual)

Pathology
— Burrowing of gravid female and larvae in jejunum cause mild or severe ulcerative jejunitis resulting in inflammatory diarrhoea or malabsorption

Symptoms
— Diarrhoea, steatorrhoea, urticaria

Treatment
— Thiabendazole with repeat course after one month

Capillaria phillipinensis **(roundworm)**

Area
— Philippines

Life cycle
— Unknown. Fish and crustacea may be secondary hosts

Symptoms
— Diarrhoea, abdominal pain, wasting, oedema and death in 2–4 months

Treatment
— Thiabendazole

Ancylostomiasis (roundworm, hookworm)

Organisms
— *Ancylostoma duodenale* or *Necator americanus*

Area
— Tropics and subtropics

Life cycle
— Adults attach to host duodenal mucosa, ingest host's blood and lay eggs to soil – hatch in 24 h to larvae (viable in soil for weeks), skin penetration to lymphatics to lungs to trachea to gut

Symptoms
— Common mild infection: symptomless
— Heavy infection: iron-deficiency anaemia

Treatment
— Mebendazole

Trichuriasis (roundworm and whipworm)

Area
— Tropics and subtropics

Life cycles
— Adults attach to mucosa in ileum and colon, lay eggs, infective state in warm moist soil after 3 weeks, ingestion, larvae in intestine mature to adults

Symptoms
— Mild infestation common: no symptoms
— Heavy infestation: dysenteric stools, weight loss, tenesmus, rectal prolapse
— Treatment mebendazole

Ascariasis (roundworm)

Area
— Tropics and subtropics

Life cycle
— Eggs ingested – hatch in small intestine, adults remain in human, eggs exit in stool

Symptoms
— Watery diarrhoea
— Heavy infection – intestinal obstruction

Treatment
— Mebendazole

Amoebiasis (protozoan, *Entamoeba histolytica*)

Area
— Worldwide but commoner in tropics and subtropics

Life cycle
— Ingestion of cysts in contaminated food and water – gastric digestion of cysts – colonisation of colon
— Factors which trigger invasion by amoebae unknown but only strains possessing certain enzymes are invasive

Symptoms
— Intermittent diarrhoea with blood and mucus resembling ulcerative colitis

Complications
— Invasion of mucosa may lead to peritoneal and liver infection with abscess formation

Diagnosis
— Cysts and amoebae in fresh warm stool
— Antibody titre of 1:128 signifies invasive infection

Treatment
— Metronidazole
— Surgery rarely needed for abscess

Giardiasis (protozoan, *Giardia lamblia*)

Area
— Worldwide but especially in areas with bad sanitation

Life cycle
— Trophozoite adheres to small intestine mucosa – cysts – contaminated water and food

Symptoms
— Commonly asymptomatic
— Common finding in protein energy malnutrition and immuno-deficiency
— May cause acute episodes of watery diarrhoea or malabsorption syndrome
— Common cause of travellers diarrhoea
— Responsible for some outbreaks of diarrhoea in day nurseries

Diagnosis
— In addition to stool examination, direct examination of duodenal aspirate or smear of duodenal mucosa has a higher success rate

Treatment
— Metronidazole

Tropical sprue

Aetiology
— Unknown
— 'Post infective' aetiology suggested by occurrence after acute gastrointestinal infection and occasional epidemics
— Some patients have overgrowth of enterobacteria in jejunum which is normally sterile
— Response to tetracycline supports an infective cause
— Sprue is comparatively rare in children which is against a simple infective mechanism

Features
— Those of malabsorption – wasting, hypoproteinaemia. Lactase deficiency frequent

Diagnosis
— Other causes of malabsorption must be excluded (gut helminths, giardiasis, coeliac disease, etc.)
— Jejunal biopsy usually shows partial villous atrophy

Treatment
— Folic acid and a good diet are usually curative
— Trimethoprim should be tried if there is no response
— (Tetracycline is standard treatment in adults but is contraindicated in children under 12 years old)

Bacterial colonisation of small intestine

Definition
— $>10^4$ colony forming units/ml jejunal fluid

Underlying causes
— Blind loops
— Stricture
— Abnormal motility
— Crohn's disease
— Previous surgery
— Short gut

Possible pathological mechanisms
— Bacterial enzymes – destruction of glycocalyx, microvilli and epithelium
— Bacterial toxins – secretion of electrolytes and water
— Deconjugation of bile salts – inhibition of absorption; morphological damage

Diagnosis
— Direct: demonstration by intubation
  NB need for excellent anaerobic techniques
— Indirect
  • Demonstration of deconjugated bile salts in jejunal fluid
  • Abnormal urinary excretion of indicans
  • Breath hydrogen analysis after lactulose or [^{14}C]glycine ingestion

Treatment
— Antibiotic therapy based on organisms isolated
— 'Blind' therapy with trimethoprim and metronidazole or similar combination
— Cholestyramine – to minimise effects of deconjugated bile salts

---

SPECIFIC DEFECTS OF ABSORPTION

Protein and amino acids

Enterokinase deficiency and trypsinogen deficiency
— Both autosomal recessive and rare
— Failure of protein digestion by trypsin occurs in both
  • Failure to thrive
  • Hypoproteinaemia and oedema
  • Steatorrhoea
— Diagnosis by pancreatic function test and demonstration of recovery of trypsin activity in juice by addition of either enterokinase or trypsinogen

Methionine malabsorption (oast house urine disease)
- Autosomal recessive
- Specific transport defect
- Clinical features:
  - Diarrhoea
  - Mental retardation
  - Convulsions
  - Hypopigmentation
- Symptoms exacerbated by methionine loading
- Improved by low methionine diet

Carbohydrate

Presentation
- Abnormal stools
  - Loose or watery
  - Frothy
  - Acidic causing perianal excoriation
- Failure to thrive

Diagnosis (see p. 178)

Glucose–galactose malabsorption
- Rare autosomal recessive disorder
- Ineffective brush border transport mechanism
- Presents in neonatal period with profuse watery diarrhoea
- Lactose, sucrose and glucose-free diet required for survival
- Carbohydrate provided as fructose

Lactose intolerance

Non-Caucasian
- Low or absent mucosal lactase is the rule in non-Caucasian individuals over the age of 5 years
- Persistence of lactase activity is dominantly inherited
- Small amounts of lactose are tolerated
- Larger amounts cause colicky abdominal pain and/or diarrhoea
- Avoid drinking milk

Secondary
- Lactase appears to be the most vulnerable brush border enzyme
- Activity is reduced after insults such as
  - Acute gastroenteritis
  - Coeliac disease in relapse
  - Gastrointestinal surgery
  - Hypoxia
  - Protein energy malnutrition
- Common cause of diarrhoea on milk-containing diets in above circumstances
- Recovery in a few days or weeks is the rule in well-nourished infants

— Use lactose-free milks but challenge regularly with lactose or ordinary milk

Congenital

— Rare autosomal recessive disorder with absent lactase activity
— Presentation similar to glucose–galactose malabsorption
— Sucrose and glucose are tolerated normally

Sucrose intolerance

— See p. 40

Fat

Abetalipoproteinaemia

Aetiology

— Absence of apoprotein results in failure of chylomicron formation

Symptoms

— Failure to thrive
— Steatorrhoea
— Later in childhood
  - Ataxia
  - Neuropathy
  - Pigmentary retinopathy
  - Cirrhosis

Diagnosis

— Acanthocytes in peripheral blood
— Low plasma cholesterol and beta-lipoprotein
— Fat soluble vitamin deficiencies
  - Undetectable vitamin E even with oral treatment
  - Use red cell peroxidase test to monitor
— Micronodular cirrhosis
— Jejunal biopsy: characteristic fat laden enterocytes

Treatment

— Low fat diet
— Vitamin E and essential fatty acids supplements prevent neurological sequelae

Vitamins

B$_{12}$ malabsorption

— See Table 13.2
— Congenital intrinsic factor (IF) deficiency
— Congenital malabsorption of IF/B$_{12}$ complex
  - Associated with proteinuria
— Distinguished by Schilling tests (p. 179)

Transcobalamin II deficiency

— Autosomal recessive
— B$_{12}$ levels normal: bound to transcobalamin I

— Megaloblastic anaemia, protracted diarrhoea
— Vitamin B_{12} (1 mg hydroxocobalamin twice weekly) IM

Folate malabsorption
— Congenital folate malabsorption may present with diarrhoea

Electrolytes

Congenital chloridorrhoea

Aetiology
— Autosomal recessively inherited defect of Cl^-/HCO_3^- exchange in ileum and colon

Clinical features
— Hydramnios in affected pregnancy
— No passage of meconium (liquid stool confused with urine)
— Abdominal distension (often confused with intestinal obstruction)
— Severe watery diarrhoea and failure to thrive
— Plasma Na^+ and K^+ and Cl^- reduced; HCO_3^- retained
— Sum of stool Na^+ and $K^+ < Cl^-$
  • Only reliable after 3 months of age

Management
— Replacement of electrolyte losses of both NaCl and KCl in approximately 1:2 ratio

Prognosis
— Normal growth and development if treated early
— Frequently brain-damaged due to late diagnosis and treatment

Defective Na^+/H^+ exchange
— Presents prenatally or in neonatal period and mimics chloride diarrhoea

Other causes of malabsorption

Congenital microvillous atrophy
— Autosomal recessive inheritance
— Presents between birth and six weeks of age
— EM of jejunal biopsy shows defective brush border and intraenterocytic brush border inclusions
— Management
  • No curative treatment
  • Support with TPN may have already started by the time of diagnosis

Autoimmune enteropathy
— Biopsy indistinguishable from coeliac disease
— Often presents before introduction of gluten
— Circulating autoantibodies including antienterocyte cytoplasm antibodies
— Some respond to hypoallergenic diet
— Some respond to steroids

CHRONIC INFLAMMATORY BOWEL DISEASE

— Crohn's disease and ulcerative colitis (UC) are considered as separate entities
— Clinically separation of large bowel Crohn's from UC may be difficult
— Crohn's disease appears to be commoner than UC in children

Crohn's disease

Incidence

— Uncommon in children but being increasingly diagnosed
  - Best estimates suggest 4–8 new child cases/year/10^6 general population in UK

Presenting features

— 1/3 childhood Crohn's present with insidious onset and non-specific features:
  - Abdominal pain (commonest)
  - Diarrhoea
  - Anorexia
  - Malaise
  - Fever
  - Growth failure
  - Delayed puberty
— Other features:
  - Rectal bleeding
  - Mouth ulcers/granulomas
  NB orofacial granulomatosis (see below)
  - Perianal ulcers
  - Perianal skin tags
  - Clubbing
  - Iritis
  - Arthritis
  NB Investigate abdominal pain and/or diarrhoea if some other feature is present, e.g. fever, anaemia, weight loss

Diagnosis

Laboratory findings

— Haematological
  - Anaemia
    - Normocytic, normochromic
    - Iron deficiency (dietary, malabsorption, blood loss)
    - Folate deficiency
    - Vitamin B_{12} deficiency
  - Leucocytosis
  - Elevated ESR and acute phase proteins

- Clinical chemistry
  - Hypoalbuminaemia (malnutrition, protein loss into gastro-intestinal tract)
  - Other abnormal liver function tests
  - Zn^{2+} and Cu^{2+} deficiency
  - Steatorrhoea (uncommon)

Radiology

- Double contrast studies are the most effective radiological technique
  - Diffuse or localised mucosal abnormality (cobblestoning) with 'skip' areas
  - Characteristic ulcer craters
  - Areas of narrowing again with 'skipping'
  - Loops of bowel separated by oedematous thickened walls
  - Fistulae
  - Rectal sparing even if large bowel involved

Colonoscopy

- Total colonoscopy with a view of the terminal ileum and multiple biopsies is probably the most sensitive diagnostic technique
  - Mucosal abnormality – pallor, 'cobblestoning'
  - Aphthous ulcers

Histology

- Classically transmucosal changes
- Oral, bowel or perianal mucosa may show characteristic non-caseating granulomata with giant cells
- May occur in macroscopically normal mucosa

Management

- Jointly between paediatric gastroenterologist and a gastrointestinal surgeon

Nutrition

- Growth failure is probably largely due to low protein energy intake
- Elemental diet (use SHS Pepdite 0–2 or 2+, Elemental 028 or similar, see Appendix B, p. 182) as a primary therapy
  - Aim to give 140% of RDA
  - For 6 weeks
  - Use overnight tube feeding with pump
  - Can go home on this regimen
- Continue high energy intake long term (e.g. 6–12 months) using dietary supplements
- Results as good as with steroids with obvious nutritional benefits in addition
- Steroids (see below)
  - May still be required for extraintestinal manifestations or colitis
  - May give additional benefits in all patients (unproven)

Drugs

— Steroids
  - Indications
    - Fever
    - Malabsorption
    - Severe and recurrent pain
    - Other moderate symptoms
    - Extraintestinal manifestations
    - Diffuse small bowel disease
    - Recurrence after surgery
  - Dosage – prednisolone 40–60 mg/m^2 for 2 weeks
  - If subjective and objective improvement (ESR, acute phase proteins, haemoglobin, albumin) reduce using a standard regimen
  - Alternate day reduction will lead to an early alternate day regimen which may be preferable in reducing complications
  - Providing that relapse does not occur then complete withdrawal should be tried. No benefit from continuous low dose steroid
— Sulphasalazine
  - Maintains steroid induced remission
  - Possible steroid sparing effect during remission
  - Dosage: 1–2 g/m^2/day
— Azothiaprine, 6-mercaptopurine and cyclosporin A have all been used for refractory patients
— Metronidazole
  - May hasten healing of abscesses and fistulae
  - 10 mg/kg/day divided doses

Surgery

— Indications
  - Disease unresponsive to medical therapy
  - Intestinal obstruction
  - Abscess
  - Fistulae
  - Haemorrhage
  - Toxic megacolon
  - Growth failure unresponsive to nutritional support
— Prognosis after surgery
  - A good initial response with an apparent remission is nearly always short lived
  - In the long term, relapse is the rule (30% in 2 years)

Prognosis

— Long periods of remission are often attainable
— May become less severe in later life
— Probably never cured

Ulcerative colitis

Incidence
— Worldwide: approximately 5/100 000 (Crohn's about 2/100 000) in developed countries; less common than Crohn's in children
— Familial: 5–10% risk in siblings of index case of chronic inflammatory bowel disease
— 14% of patients present in childhood

In infancy
— Indistinguishable histologically from classical UC
— Probably >90% associated with food protein intolerance
  • Manage at least initially as protein intolerance
— Prognosis good (as for protein intolerance rather than UC)

Presenting features
— Change in bowel habit – diarrhoea, blood, mucus and pus, especially at night
— Rectal bleeding
— Tenesmus (occasional)
— Abdominal pain
— Growth retardation – late feature compared with Crohn's
— Extraintestinal
  • Fever
  • Erythema nodosum
  • Pauciarticular arthritis especially sacroiliitis
  • Uveitis
  • Disordered liver function
  • Chronic active hepatitis
  • Ankylosing spondylitis (associated with HLA B27 tissue type)
  • Pyoderma gangrenosum (rare)

Diagnosis
Radiology
— Changes start distally with variable extent proximally
— Affected bowel does not contain faecal material, giving a clue to extent of disease
— Double contrast enema shows loss of motility, loss of haustral pattern and an abnormal mucosal pattern with crypt ulcers
— Normal barium follow through makes Crohn's less likely

Endoscopy
— Mandatory since radiology may be normal in presence of disease
  • Reddening of mucosa
  • Obliteration of vascular pattern
  • Contact bleeding
  • Superficial ulcers
  • Pseudopolyps – islands of normal mucosa surrounded by granulation tissue

Histology
— Several biopsies should be obtained from different parts of the colon even if macroscopically normal

- Mucosal infiltration with lymphocytes, plasma cells and eosinophils
- Congestion and haemorrhages
- Goblet cell depletion
- Loss of orientation of mucosal glands
- Crypt abscesses

Differential diagnosis
— Crohn's colitis
— Acute infective colitis (*Campylobacter*, etc.)
— Amoebiasis
— Cow's milk protein intolerance (especially in infants)
— Other protein intolerance (e.g. soy)

Management
Drugs
— Ulcerative proctitis
  - Steroid enemas
  - Colifoam with sulphasalazine enemas
  - Cromoglycate may have a place in therapy
— Distal disease (not beyond splenic flexure)
  - Steroid Colifoam enemas
  - Oral sulphasalazine or equivalent
— More extensive disease
  - Systemic steroids in addition (1–2 mg/kg for 2 weeks)
— Tail off slowly
  - Restart if relapse occurs and tail off more slowly

Nutrition
— Repair of fluid, electrolyte and albumin deficits may be essential first line therapy
— Thereafter adequate nutrition is important and supplementary enteral feed (see Appendix B, p. 182) may be helpful

Surgery
— Indications
  - Toxic megacolon and no response to medical treatment
  - Chronic disease
    - Steroid dependence
    - Growth failure
    - Delayed puberty
    - School absence
    - >10 years active (controlled) disease
  - Colonic perforation
  - Local complications
  - Extraintestinal complications
— Usually a total colectomy
  - May be combined with excision of rectal mucosa and retention of rectum as faecal reservoir (Soave)

Complications

Acute presentation or relapse
- >5 bowel actions/24 h
- Grossly bloody stool
- Pyrexia >37.8°C
- Tachycardia >90
- Haemoglobin falling
- Plasma albumin <30 g/l

Toxic megacolon
— Usually during a relapse rather than at first presentation
— Diagnosed if >4 of following clinical features
  NB All features masked by steroid therapy
  - As for acute relapse and in addition
  - Prostration
  - Vomiting
  - Abdominal distension
  - Diffuse abdominal tenderness
  - Diminished bowel sounds
  - Plain X-ray – colonic dilatation with gas
— Management
  - Bed rest
  - Continuous nasogastric drainage/suction
  - Parenteral nutrition
  - Parenteral steroids (IV prednisolone)
  - Twice daily X-ray to exclude perforation
  NB Barium studies are **contraindicated** (risk of perforation)
— Surgery
  - Immediate for perforation
  - After 48–72 h intensive medical treatment with no major clinical improvement
  - Colectomy and ileostomy with subsequent Soave procedure
— Prognosis
  - Mortality is 5–30% and greater if surgery is required after 48 h

Malignancy
— Is an important risk in adult life
  - Action necessary after 10 years disease
— Management
  - With advent of Soave procedure elective colectomy may be preferable to
  - Annual or biannual colonoscopy and biopsies after the first decade
  - Colectomy for carcinoma *in situ*

Prognosis
— Remitting disease but usually chronic
— Onset at <2 years carries a poor prognosis (excluding that due to cow's milk protein intolerance, etc.)

— Colectomy results in permanent cure
— Rectal mucosal excision is required to remove risk of malignancy
— Ileorectal anastomosis takes child through puberty: most patients eventually revert to ileostomy unless they have a Soave procedure
— Ulcerative proctitis carries good prognosis of complete recovery after 6–12 months

6 FAILURE TO THRIVE WITHOUT OBVIOUS GASTROINTESTINAL SYMPTOMS

Patients referred

— Infants who fail to gain weight at the expected rate
  - See percentile charts, e.g. Tanner and Whitehouse, Castlemead Publications, Hertford, UK
— Children below the third centile for height or weight
— Children whose parents claim they have not gained or have lost weight over a period

Definition of failure to thrive

— Diagnosis based on serial measurements, over a significant period (e.g. 1–3 months in infancy; 6–12 months in older children)
  - Actual weight loss
  - Static weight or height
  - Serial measurements height and/or weight crossing centiles in a downward direction
— Height or weight more than 3 standard deviations below the mean (−3 SD)
  - −2 SD is approximated by distance between 50th and 3rd centiles
— Weight less than 80% of 50th centile weight
  - This is an international definition used in studies of nutritional status; <80% = severe malnutrition; <60% = marasmus)
— Weight for height more than 3 SD below the mean for age
  - e.g. using Cole's slide rule (Castlemead Publications, Hertford, UK) or tables

Aetiology

— In the UK less than half of the children fulfilling a definition of failure to thrive will have an organic cause other than poor dietary intake

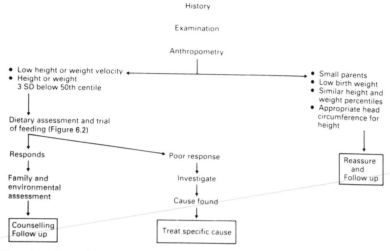

Figure 6.1 Failure to thrive

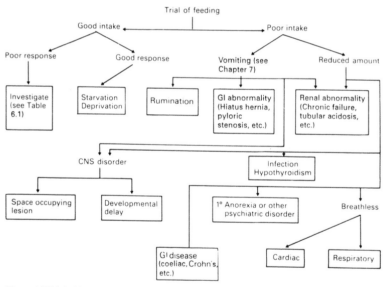

Figure 6.2 Trial of feeding

Management

— See Figures 6.1 and 6.2

History

— Family history of short stature
— Heights of parents and siblings
— Pregnancy history particularly in relation to possible congenital
infections

— Birth history including gestation, birth weight and, if possible, length and head circumference.
NB Newborn length usually unreliable
— Weight during the first year is often available from infant welfare clinic records
— Systems enquiry
  • Developmental progress
  • Exercise intolerance or breathlessness
  • Abdominal pain or headache
  • Vomiting (including posseting) or diarrhoea
  • Frequency, dysuria or polydipsia
— Dietary assessment assisted by a dietitian
— Social report (family practitioner, health visitor, social worker)

Examination
— Check measurements personally

Newborns
— Constitutional small stature is suggested by an infant being light for gestational age who is also short with a small head circumference
— Causes include:
  • Small parents
  • Genetic disorders
    – Chromosomal, e.g. Down, Turner, etc.
    – Dysmorphic, e.g. Russell–Silver
    – Skeletal, e.g. osteodystrophy
  • Intrauterine infections, e.g. rubella, toxoplasma, CMV
  • Intrauterine insults
    – Fetal alcohol syndrome
    – Fetal phenytoin syndrome
    – etc.
— Nutritional causes of light for dates infants affect length less than weight, and head circumference less than either
— Causes include:
  • Gestational hypertension
  • Maternal starvation
  • Placental insufficiency
  • Maternal smoking

Infants and children
— Infants with nutritional causes of light for dates tend to show rapid catch up growth
— Infants with constitutional causes usually follow below but parallel to normal centiles
— Longtitudinal data is invaluable and may show a 'dropping off' the previous centile while still being within normal range
— Growth velocity charts allow accurate plotting of growth velocities
  • All measurements should be made personally

- Less than 6 month intervals of plotting may give erroneous results
— Parental height
  - Centiles for the child based on parental height are published as separate charts (Castlemead Publications, Hertford, UK)
  - Useful estimates may be made using only standard growth charts
  - At adult range of chart (18 or 19 years) mark 'mid-parental height prediction'
    - Plot parent's height of the same sex on the child's chart
    - Plot other parent's height after correction for difference between sexes
    - Add 13 cm (5 in) to mother's height for a boy and subtract 13 cm (5 in) from father's height for a girl
    - Then plot 'mid-parental' height prediction at point midway between parents' plots
  - 95% limits for children's adult heights are then 8.5 cm (3.5 in) either side of this midparental prediction
    - Thus define 3rd and 97th centiles on the population chart for this particular family

Assessment of anthropometric data
— Knowledge of weight, height, sitting height, head circumference and skinfold thickness centiles enables a reasonable guess as to possible causes
— Nutritional failure to thrive including gastrointestinal disease
  - Tends to cause a greater diminution in weight and skinfold than in height or in head circumference
— Endocrine causes including growth hormone deficiency or hypothyroidism
  - Tend to affect height more than weight or skinfold
— In growth hormone deficiency
  - Weight is usually greater than 50th centile for height and skinfold rarely less than 25th centile
— Constitutional and metabolic causes usually result in an equivalent reduction of growth potential in height and weight
— Emotional deprivation may result in the classical features of either nutritional or endocrine failure to thrive
— Specific CNS dysfunction may be associated with a disproportionate head circumference – either large or small
— In bone disorders sitting height may be relatively normal compared with short standing height

General physical examination
— Look for dysmorphic features which may suggest a specific diagnosis
— Look for other evidence of deprivation, neglect or abuse
— Systems examination may reveal chronic cardiorespiratory or renal disease etc.

Trial of feeding

— Many authorities recommend this before or associated with specific investigation (see Figure 6.2)
— Hospital admission is often necessary in order to establish dietary intake
— Dietary intake should be above that recommended for age and preferably 40% above that to constitute an adequate test
— Increased weight velocity will be virtually immediate if dietary insufficiency is the cause
  ● May be delayed by 2–4 weeks if there is severe emotional deprivation
— Procedure is threatening to parents and needs tactful handling

Failed trial

— Failure to achieve adequate intake
  ● Psychosomatic cause, e.g. behavioural disorder
  ● Chronic debilitating disease, e.g. renal failure
— Occurrence of gastrointestinal symptoms
  ● Vomiting, e.g. hiatus hernia
  ● Diarrhoea, e.g. coeliac, cystic fibrosis
  ● Abdominal distension, e.g. malrotation
  ● Abdominal pain, e.g. Crohn's
— No weight gain in spite of good intake and apparent good positive balance of energy intake
  ● Other system disorder, e.g. cardiac, renal, metabolic, chronic infection, endocrine, emotional
  ● Constitutional small stature
  ● Recorded intake not going in

Table 6.1 Investigations for failure to thrive

Investigation	Disorder(s)
Haemoglobin	Malabsorption/malnutrition
RBC folate	
Alkaline phosphatase	
White cell differential	Immunodeficiency
Immunoglobulins	
Electrolytes	Chronic renal failure
Urea	
Creatinine	
Calcium	
Phosphate	
pH (serum and urine)	Renal tubular acidosis
Microurine	Urinary tract infection
Transaminases	Liver disease
Stool microscopy	Giardiasis
Chromatography	Carbohydrate intolerance
Jejunal biopsy	Coeliac disease
Barium follow through	Congenital anomaly, Crohn's disease

Successful trial

— Previous inadequate dietary intake
  - Poor socioeconomic situation
  - Poor management of family diet
  - Behaviour disorder
  - Neglect
— Emotional deprivation
  - Often difficult to diagnose clinically and requires psychosocial investigation to exclude

Further investigation

— If above procedure has been followed a specific area of investigation will be indicated (see Table 6.1)
— Is outside the scope of this book, covering a wide area of paediatrics

7 FEEDING PROBLEMS AND VOMITING

DISORDERED SWALLOWING

Aetiology

Immaturity
— Swallowing is a complex voluntary and reflex process
— Begins at about 16 weeks gestation
— Mature and reliable at about 34 weeks gestation
— Good prognosis in absence of other neurological abnormality

Anatomical abnormality
— Micrognathia (Pierre Robin sequence)
— Macroglossia
— Severe tongue tie
— Small palatal cleft
— Submucous cleft palate

Neurological dysfunction
— Common in cerebral palsy of any type
— Bulbar or pseudobulbar palsies
— Moebius syndrome – congenital cranial nerve nuclear agenesis
  • Usually sporadic, occasionally dominant
  • Disorder of eye movement and/or closure is a constant feature
  • Facial muscle involvement common
  • Palate tongue and lips may be involved giving rise to dysphagia
— Familial dysautonomia
  • Autosomal recessive in Ashkenazi Jews
  • Severe swallowing difficulty from infancy
  • Cyanotic attacks and bronchopneumonia
  • Variable mental retardation
  • Absent corneal reflex and tears
  • Indifference to painful stimuli
  • Poor control of blood pressure and body temperature

- Intradermal histamine (0.05 ml of 1/1000 solution) produces no flare
  - Use a control for comparison
- Methacholine eye drops restore the absent corneal reflex
- Management directed towards active treatment of chest infection and protection of the cornea

Diagnosis

— Experienced personnel are required for each technique
— Observation of swallowing pattern
— Listening (with a stethoscope) to the pattern of swallowing
— Direct observation by nasal endoscope
— Cine or video swallow of radio contrast
— Objective assessment by measurement of timing of respiration and components of the suck/swallow sequence
  - Exeter Dysphagia Assessment Technique (EDAT)

Management

— A period of tube feeding may allow maturation to occur
— An improved pattern of feeding may be established by trial and error
— In cerebral palsy propping the child upright facing the mother and spoon feeding (taking care to hold the spoon in the midline) may help
— Palatal appliances may be invaluable in specific situations

Disordered oesophageal transit

Aetiology

Without stricture

— Common after repair of tracheo-oesophageal fistulae
— Achalasia
  - Food fails to pass through the cardia
  - Accumulates in a dilated redundant oesophagus
  - Frequently spills over into the trachea
  - May present as anorexia nervosa
  - Contrast radiology may not be diagnostic initially
— Familial dysautonomia (see above)

Intrinsic stricture

— With gastro-oesophageal reflux
— After corrosive burns
— After tracheo-oesophageal fistula repair

Extrinsic compression

— Duplication cysts
— Mediastinal mass
— Vascular 'rings', etc.

Diagnosis

— By cine or video contrast radiology

VOMITING, REFLUX, ETC.

— Vomiting
  • Posseting
  • Rumination
  • Regurgitation/gastro-oesophageal reflux
  • True vomiting

Posseting

— Regurgitation of small amounts of liquid food after feeds
— Stains rather than soaks clothing and sheets
— Does not cause failure to thrive
— Considered normal

Rumination

— Regurgitation of small amounts of food into the mouth which is then 'chewed' with apparent self-gratification
— Rare disorder which may be familial

Regurgitation/gastro-oesophageal reflux

— Larger amounts of liquid food are vomited between feeds
— Volumes are large enough to soak clothes and bedding
— Food lost may be grossly exaggerated or underestimated in the history
— Failure to thrive may result
— Common disorder in infancy
— Reflux may be demonstrated by contrast radiology or scintiscan or oesophageal pH monitoring (p. 172)

Management

— Diagnosis may be made on the basis of history
— Precise anatomical diagnosis not necessary (see Hiatus hernia below)
— If no failure to thrive explain mechanism to parents and give good prognosis
— Propping upright after feeds for 60 to 90 minutes may be sufficient
  • A rigid 'baby relax' chair is needed rather than a hammock type
  • Longer periods, e.g. all day or even 24 h propping may be necessary
— Thickening of bottle or expressed breast milk feeds (to a good custard consistency)
  • Use low energy carbohydrate agent such as Carobel

— Gaviscon (infant or sachet) given after feeds is effective
  • Na^+ content of 2 mmol/2 g sachet restricting its use in young infants
  • Useful in breast-fed infants

In small infants

— The optimum posture is prone with head of cot elevated 30° and baby in a sling
— For those that do not respond a period of nasogastric or nasoduodenal tube feeding may be necessary

Prognosis

— Most resolve spontaneously in early infancy
— Symptoms lessen markedly when the infant is sitting independently
— Nearly all are resolved by the time the child is walking or learns to swallow regurgitated feed
— See below for complications

Hiatus hernia and complicated gastro-oesophageal reflux

— True or sliding hiatus hernia is often difficult to distinguish from simple regurgitation
  • May be associated with a malrotation
— Prognosis for spontaneous resolution of hiatus hernia symptoms is good
— Free reflux or hiatus hernia may result in complications
  • Failure to thrive
  • Occult blood loss and anaemia
  • Pain from oesophagitis
  • Stricture
  • Aspiration
    – May occur subclinically
    – May be a rare cause of apnoeic cot death
    – Presenting with recurrent chest infection
    – 24 h oesophageal pH monitoring may be useful (p. 172)
    – Examine bronchial lavage aspirate for fat laden macrophages
    – Scintigraphic studies with labelled feeds
— Presence of complications such as pain or blood loss necessitate endoscopic assessment of therapy
— H_2 antagonists aid healing of oesophagitis
  • Increase dose until fasting gastric pH >4
— Also consider nasoduodenal feeding, antacids, Gaviscon, sucralfate, cisapride, etc.
— Operation (usually Nissen fundoplication) is rarely required
  • Failure to respond to medical treatment
  • Stricture
  • Severe aspiration

TRUE VOMITING

— Forceful regurgitation of most of the contents of the stomach at one time
— Evidence of duodenogastric reflex shown by bile staining

Aetiology

— Causes arranged chronologically in Table 7.1 with emphasis on the neonatal period

Diagnosis

— See Table 7.1

Presentation in the neonatal period

— On the first day must be distinguished from regurgitation of a tracheo-oesophageal fistula (see p. 5)
— Anatomical obstruction is considered early
  • Pass nasogastric tube
  • Inject 10 ml of air
  • Take erect and supine X-rays
  • Distribution of air fluid levels may establish diagnosis
— If no apparent obstruction
  • Investigate for infection
  • Consider cerebral causes
  • Consider galactosaemia
  • Consider and investigate other possible metabolic causes, e.g. organic acidaemias, hyperammonaemias
— Regurgitation is a diagnosis of exclusion but may be confirmed by effect of posture

With drowsiness

  • Consider meningitis, septicaemia
— If in doubt: culture and treat
  • Consider raised intracranial pressure
  • Look for other evidence of trauma
  • Metabolic causes
— Hyperventilation suggests acidosis
  • Check blood sugar
    – Low in Reye's, urea cycle defects, galactosaemia
    – High in diabetes mellitus
  • Check blood gas
  • Check electrolytes/or anion gap – organic acidaemia
— Hypotension
  • Adrenal crisis
  • Severe dehydration
  • Malaria

With diarrhoea

  • Gastroenteritis
  • Food poisoning
  • Partial intestinal obstruction

Table 7.1 Causes of vomiting

First day of life	
Alimentary tract obstruction	Duodenal atresia
	Jejunal atresia
	Malrotation/volvulus
	Diaphragmatic hernia
	Duplications
Incompetent cardiac sphincter	Hiatus hernia
	Simple incompetence
Cerebral	Birth trauma
	Raised intracranial pressure
Metabolic	Galactosaemia
Infections	Meningitis
	Septicaemia
First week of life	
As above plus:	
Alimentary tract obstruction	Meconium ileus
	Hirschsprung's disease
	Milk plug
	Functional obstruction
	Anal atresia
	Strangulated hernia
	Intussusception
Metabolic	Hyperammonaemias
	Organic acidaemias
	Hypercalcaemia
	Adrenocorticoid deficiency
Infections	Gastritis
	Gastroenteritis
	Otitis media
Dietetic	Cow's milk protein intolerance
After the first week of life	
Most of the above plus:	
Alimentary tract obstruction	Pyloric stenosis (hypertrophic)
	Appendicitis
	Foreign body/ascariasis
	Peptic ulceration
	Bezoar
Metabolic	Diabetic ketoacidosis
	Drug ingestion/overdose
	Reye's syndrome
Infections	Infectious fevers
	Malaria
	Infectious hepatitis
	Sinusitis
Dietetic	Overeating
	Indiscretion
	Food poisoning
	Coeliac disease
Other	Motion sickness
	Periodic syndrome
	Cyclical vomiting

- Acute ileocolitis, e.g. in UC or Hirschsprung's
- Appendicitis

With chronic abdominal pain
- Peptic ulcer

Other causes
- Infections
  - Epidemic fevers
  - Infectious hepatitis
  - Urinary tract infection
  - Otitis media and sinusitis
- Paralytic ileus
- Drug abuse
- Cyclical vomiting/periodic syndrome
- Vestibulitis
- Motion sickness
- Overeating, bulimia, indiscretion

Hypertrophic pyloric stenosis

Incidence
- 3 per 1000 liveborn infants
- Male to female ratio 4:1
- Commoner
  - In firstborns especially boys
  - With a family history (especially maternal)
  - In Caucasians
  - In a number of apparently unrelated disorders (Table 7.2)

Table 7.2 Conditions in which hypertrophic pyloric stenosis is more common

Partial thoracic stomach
Oesophageal atresia
Rubella embryopathy
Turner syndrome
Trisomy 18
Long arm deletion 21
Smith–Lemli–Opitz syndrome
Cornelia de Lange syndrome
Phenylketonuria
Maternal myasthenia gravis
Thalidomide embryopathy
Blood group O or B

Clinical features
- Vomiting usually begins between third and eighth weeks
  - Gradually increasing severity
  - Develops characteristic projectile nature
  - Baby usually only vomits once between feeds, rather than continuously, as in regurgitation

— Examination during feed shows
  • Visible waves of peristalsis moving from left to right and downwards in left hypochondrium
  • Palpable tumour in area in between liver and rectus abdominis in the right hypochondrium
  • Tumour is variable in size and consistency even in the same infant as pyloric muscle contracts and relaxes
— Persistent severe vomiting results in
  • Constipation
  • Hyponatraemia, hypokalaemia, hypochloraemia and alkalosis
  • Dehydration occurs late

Diagnosis

— Clinical and biochemical features as above
— Imaging can be helpful
  • Investigator needs experience
  • Ultrasound can be used to show hypertrophied pylorus as compared with standard measurements
  • Contrast studies show gastric outlet obstruction with classical 'double bracket' sign

Management

— Measure acid–base status and plasma electrolytes
— Calculate sodium deficit (bodyweight in kg × 0.6 × [135 − plasma Na^+] add normal requirements (2.5 mmol/kg) and replace with saline over 24 h
  • Calculation of chloride deficit may be preferable (bodyweight in kg × 0.6 × [100 − plasma Cl^-])
  • This allows for hypochloraemia of acid loss
  NB It is unnecessary to correct alkalosis except by NaCl administration
  NB Operation is not urgent and the infant's biochemistry should be normal before submission to surgery
— Ramstedt's pyloromyotomy is usually straightforward and may be done under local if preferred, e.g. if anaesthetic cover poor
— 'Medical' management with atropine methonitrate (Eumydrin) has no place in routine management
— Breast or bottle-feeding may be begun after full recovery from the anaesthetic at 12–24 h. Regrading is probably of no value
— Small amounts of vomiting postoperatively may be ignored
  NB Regurgitation with short oesophagus is sometimes associated

Cyclical vomiting

— Term reserved for recurrent episodes of severe, 'non-organic' vomiting
  NB Consider organic causes of recurrent vomiting
  • Intermittent obstruction

- Metabolic disorder, e.g. urea cycle defect
— Distinguished from recurrent abdominal pain syndrome with vomiting
— Usually occurs in children with significant psychopathology
— Episodes may result in severe dehydration and/or metabolic disturbance which can be life threatening
— Episode may build up gradually or start acutely
— Associated craving for fluids perpetuates the symptoms
— Emergency management is directed to rehydration and metabolic correction
— Episodes may be aborted by chlorpromazine
— Psychiatric management in selected children
— Resolves with standard supportive methods in the majority (see pp. 30, 104)

OTHER FEEDING PROBLEMS

Infantile colic

— Loosely defined disturbance of early infancy
— Affects more than 1 in 10 infants

Features

— Periods of excessive irritability and apparent abdominal pain associated with drawing up of the legs
— Episodes usually related to feeding occurring in the latter half of a feed and resulting in its termination
— Characteristically worse in the afternoon and evening
— Episodes of pain often accompanied by borborygmi + flatus PR
— Commonly remits by three months but by no means always
— Occurs in bottle-fed or breast-fed infants
— Association with 'worrying' mothers may be a secondary rather than a causative one

Management

— Referral to hospital usually result of
  - Prolonged history
  - Excessively worried parents
  - Apparently severe pain
  - Failure to thrive associated with low intake
— Consider other causes of crying
  - Hunger/thirst, e.g. insufficient breast milk, too small feeds
  - Learnt behavioural response
  - Infection, e.g. urinary tract infection, otitis
— Simple reassurance in a well, thriving infant may allow natural remission in time

— Dicyclomine hydrochloride (Merbentyl) (5 mg 20 minutes before feeds) is often effective
  • Now withdrawn from British National Formulary for this indication
  • Overdosage by parents was common
— Some respond to withdrawal of cow's milk from their diet (and mother's diet if breast feeding)
  • Cow's milk protein intolerance and lactose intolerance have been demonstrated in some infants with colic

Food refusal and food fads

Aetiological factors

— Weaning is an important milestone of normal psychological development and is often resisted by the infant
— Failure of parental persistence in offering weaning foods allow the infant to gain control
— Overestimation of nutritional requirements of infants and toddlers causes parents to offer attractive alternatives when food is refused

Management

— Reassurance that starvation is unlikely to supervene
— Lessening of overt parental concern may result in the child eating more
— Restriction of food intake to meal times
— Parents eating at the same time as the child
— Reward for good eating by favourite foods being offered **after** satisfactory meals

Prognosis

— Usually but not invariably excellent
— Occasionally, children continue to have a very low intake in spite of above simple measures and require psychological intervention

8 GASTROINTESTINAL BLEEDING

Presentation

Severity

— Massive bleeding with circulatory collapse
— Intermittent with history of melaena etc.
— Chronic (occult) giving rise to anaemia
— Subclinical causing no symptoms

Site

— Often difficult to establish at presentation
— Coffee grounds or fresh haematemesis, always upper gastro-intestinal bleeding
— Small amounts of fresh blood per rectum indicate lower gastrointestinal bleeding
— Streaking of stools indicates rectal or anal bleeding

Aetiology

— Exclude swallowed blood
  NB In neonates use Apt test to exclude maternal blood
— Many disorders cause upper or lower tract bleeding or both (see Table 8.1)
  NB Massive bleeds usually originate in the upper gastro-intestinal tract
— Enterocolitis may produce massive bleeding but usually as a late manifestation

Table 8.1 Differential diagnosis of gastrointestinal bleeding in children

Upper and/or lower tract bleeding

Blood disorder	Idiopathic thrombocytopenic purpura
	Blood dyscrasia
	Disseminated intravascular coagulation
	Congenital bleeding disorders,
	e.g. factor VIII deficiency
Vascular disorders	Haemangioma
	Hereditary telangiectasis
	Vasculitis, e.g. collagen disorders
	Ehlers Danlos syndrome
Anomalies	Duplications
Neoplasm	Polyps (single, multiple, Peutz Jeghers)
Mechanical	Foreign body

Upper tract bleeding

Pseudo	Swallowed blood
Peptic	Oesophagitis
	Acute gastritis
	Gastric ulcer
	Duodenal ulcer
	Stress
Mechanical	Mallory–Weiss
Vascular	Varices
	Malformations

Lower tract bleeding

Inflammatory	Ulcerative colitis
	Crohn's disease
	Allergy, e.g. Cow's milk, soya
	Entercolitis
	Necrotising
	Bacterial
	Pseudomembranous
	Radiation
Anomalies	Meckel's diverticulum
Vascular	Haemorrhoids
Mechanical	Varices
	Volvulus
	Intussusception
	Anal fissure
	Rectal prolapse

NB Massive bleeds usually originate in the upper GI tract. Enterocolitis may produce massive bleeding but usually as a late manifestation.

MANAGEMENT OF LARGE BLEEDS

— Resuscitation precedes investigation
— Immediate transfusion is required for a shocked patient
 • Use whole blood, plasma, plasma expanders or normal saline in a rapid infusion of 10–30 ml/kg

— Monitoring of colloid and fluid requirements by a central venous pressure line is mandatory
— Rising pulse or falling blood pressure give late confirmation of transfusion requirements
— Overtransfusion results in an increased risk of continuing bleeding or rebleeding as well as risks of pulmonary oedema, etc.

Diagnosis

History and examination
— Joint undertaking by physician, surgeon and radiologist
— Evidence of swallowed blood from inspection of the nose and part of the nasal space
— History of
  - Previous episodes suggests a vascular lesion
  - Pain suggests a peptic lesion
  - Vomiting suggests Mallory–Weiss syndrome
— Signs of portal venous hypertension/cirrhosis
  - Hepatosplenomegaly
  - Jaundice
  - Large abdominal veins
  - Haemorrhoids
  - Ascites and oedema
  - Spider naevi, liver nails and palms
— Evidence of bleeding diathesis
  - Bleeding from other sites (e.g. venepunctures) and specimens not clotting
— Skin manifestations of underlying disorder
  - Peutz–Jeghers syndrome, familial polyposis
  - Hereditary telangiectasis
  - Ehlers–Danlos syndrome
— Abdominal signs suggesting a ruptured viscus or enterocolitis

Investigation
— Coagulation studies and platelets (repeat after massive blood transfusion)
— Passage of nasogastric tube and gastric wash out may confirm gastric/oesophageal rather than post pyloric bleeding
— X-rays may demonstrate a mass, evidence of perforation, intestinal obstruction or enterocolitis
— Plasma urea/creatinine ratio helps to distinguish
  - Dehydration – ratio high
  - Renal failure – ratio normal
  - Excessive protein metabolism – ratio high

Special techniques
- May enable confirmation of the site of bleeding prior to laparotomy
- Barium contrast studies of limited value
  - May demonstrate presence of abnormality, e.g. varices which are not bleeding
- Upper and lower gastrointestinal endoscopy of proven value in adults
- Angiography during an acute bleed is occasionally the only helpful test
- [^{99}Te] pertechnate scanning for ectopic mucosa (Meckel's diverticulum)
- See confirmation and investigation of blood loss
- See management of the problem bleeder

Varices

- Successful management requires an expert team approach
- Confirmation by endoscopy or contrast studies
- Avoid over transfusion by keeping central venous pressure at 1–3 cmH$_2$O
- Institute appropriate treatment for prevention of hepatic encephalopathy (see p. 132)
- Pass a soft 8 or 10 FR gauge nasogastric tube and aspirate every few minutes
  - Allows monitoring of blood loss
  - Prevents further blood passing into intestine
  - Measure gastric pH
- Give H$_2$ blocker (e.g. Cimetidine IV 20 mg/kg/day initially) to keep gastric pH >4
- Give either
  - Vasopressin, dose 0.4 u/1.73 m^2/min
    - Add 200 units to 500 ml of 5% dextrose
    - Give 1 ml/1.73 m^2/min
  - Glypressin (= triglycyl lysine vasopressin)
    - Dose = 2 mg IV 6-hourly
    - Produces
    - Abdominal cramps
    - Pallor
    - Defecation
- Locate appropriate size Sengstaken–Blakemore tube or equivalent and an experienced user
  - Use is indicated if
    - Blood loss exceeds replaceable rate
    - Failure of above management after 12–24 h

- Oesophageal balloon may not be required. Try effect of gastric balloon and traction only first, thus reducing considerably the complications
- Check tube position by X-ray
- Observe for cardiac or respiratory embarrassment
- Deflate oesophageal balloon regularly if used
- After 24h without bleeding relax traction and deflate balloons
— After further 24h without bleeding – remove
— Avoid surgery if at all possible
  - Operative mortality is high
  - Cause and rational treatment cannot be established in the acute situation
  - A long postponement is a considerable advantage in the growing child
— Transhepatic or endoscopic injection of sclerosing agents are increasingly used techniques
  - Emergency portasystemic shunting very high mortality
  - Staple-gun oesophageal transection safer
  - Elective porto-systemic shunt
    - Technically difficult to maintain shunt patency <8 years of age
    - Variable incidence of encephalopathy

Lower tract bleeding

— Less common in children
— Usually with other serious disorder, e.g. enterocolitis
— Occasionally due to vascular malformation
— General management as for upper tract bleeding
  - Contrast studies contraindicated in acute colitis
  - Endoscopy desirable
  - Angiography occasionally useful

Management after recovery

— Most bleeds resolve with medical management
— Contrast radiology has a greater role than in acute phase
— Endoscopy remains important
— Angiography usually unrewarding
— Assessment of degree and site of lesion causing portal hypertension and liver function
— If no cause found with above investigations await events. Many bleeds do not recur
  NB Forbid **any** salicylate

MANAGEMENT OF THE PROBLEM BLEEDER

— More than one severe bleed for which no cause can be found
— Carefully carried out contrast studies
  - Duodenal enema with direct introduction of barium into the duodenum for the upper series
  - Double contrast for lower studies
— Upper and lower endoscopy
— [^{99}Te] pertechnate gamma scan
  - Early picture may detect flush in an arteriovenous malformation
  - Standard timed pictures to detect concentration in ectopic gastric mucosa in a Meckel's diverticulum
— Gamma scan using ^{99}Te-labelled red cells
  - While bleeding
  - Less invasive than angiography
— Selective angiography
— Ultimately laparotomy and if necessary operative endoscopy threading the endoscope along the whole small bowel

Peptic lesions

— Massive bleeding from peptic ulcer rare in childhood
— Stress ulcers associated with
  - Raised intracranial pressure
  - Burns
  - Steroids
  - Salicylate
— Acute gastritis may cause severe haemorrhage
— Management is usually medical
  - Nasogastric suction
  - Antacids
  - H_2 blockers (see under Varices, p. 92)
— No evidence of benefit for treatment of bleeding: may hasten healing
— Surgery
  - Only if exact diagnosis is established
  - Or bleeding is uncontrollable

Vascular malformation/perforation of vessel by foreign body

— Confirmation by angiography
— Resuscitation before surgery

Bleeding disorders

— Treat as appropriate
  - Platelet transfusion
  - Fresh frozen plasma
  - Specific factor concentrates
  - Vitamin K

Polyposis

— Generalised juvenile polyposis, familial polyposis coli or Peutz–Jeghers syndrome may all present with episodes of gastrointestinal bleeding
— Juvenile polyps of the colon
  - Commonest
  - Isolated
  - Pedunculated
  - Hamartomatous
  - Rarely familial
  - No tendency to malignancy
— Familial adenomatous polyposis coli
  - Family history – autosomal dominant
  - Multiple polyps on sigmoidoscopy or on contrast studies
  - Lesions are premalignant adenomata
  - Management is surgical with colectomy and ileostomy or ileoproctostomy with removal of rectal mucosa and a pull through (Soave)
  - Unaffected relatives should have yearly colonoscopy – surgical management if lesions identified
— Peutz–Jeghers syndrome
  - Family history – autosomal dominant
  - Mucocutaneous pigmented spots on lips, face and fingers
  - Polyps throughout the gastrointestinal tract
  - Benign hamartomata
  - Management is expectant reserving surgery for removal of polyps causing excessive bleeding or intussusception
— Generalised juvenile polyposis
  - Polyps contain mucin retention cysts
  - Management as for Peutz–Jeghers
  - GI malignancy risk is increased

Rectal bleeding

— Small quantities of frank blood passed per rectum either with or without faeces
— Proctoscopy should be done routinely
— Usually associated with
  - Rectal polyp

- Rectal prolapse
- Anal fissure
- Haemorrhoids
— All managed conservatively
— Less often in ulcerative proctitis (see p. 70) or Crohn's disease (see p. 66)

MANAGEMENT OF OCCULT GASTROINTESTINAL BLOOD LOSS

Presentation
— Anaemia
— Failure to thrive
— Other gastrointestinal symptoms
Aetiology
— May include most disorders listed in Table 8.1
Commoner causes
— Reflux oesophagitis
— Anatomical abnormalities (e.g. duplication)
— Inflammatory bowel disease
— Amoebiasis (not common in UK)
— Gastrointestinal allergy, e.g. cow's milk protein intolerance
— Ileocolic anastamoses
— Meat based diets (e.g. comminuted chicken) in infants may give false positives on screening tests
Confirmation
— Amidopyrine tests are the most reliable in childhood
— Weak positives (only positive with 20% amidopyrine) are not usually clinically significant
— 'Faecatwin' distinguishes human haemoglobin from contaminants in stool
Investigation
— Quantitation of loss
  - Stool testing
  - Haemoglobin and film
  - Serum iron and total iron binding capacity/ferritin
  - ^{51}Cr-labelled red cell studies
Management
— Treatment of cause if established
— Possible trial of cow's milk free diet in infants
— Iron supplements if no cause established
  - Keep under observation during and after iron therapy

9 PROTEIN-LOSING ENTEROPATHY

Physiological protein loss

— Some serum protein passes into the gastrointestinal tract
— Probably less than 10% of total protein catabolised by this route
— IgA actively secreted
— Albumin and other serum proteins probably leak into lumen in association with loss of villous tip cells

Aetiology of excessive loss

Table 9.1 Causes of protein losing enteropathy

Stomach
    Hypertrophic 'gastritis' (Menetrier's disease)
    Eosinophilic gastroenteritis
    Trichobezoar

Small intestine
    Intestinal lymphangiectasia
    Coeliac disease
    Crohn's disease
    Tropical sprue
    Eosinophilic gastroenteritis
    Tuberculosis
    Lymphosarcoma
    Hookworm
    Henoch–Schönlein purpura
    Kwashiorkor
    Giardiasis
    Malrotation/volvulus
    Intestinal stasis/partial obstruction/blind loop

Large intestine
    Ulcerative colitis
    Crohn's disease
    Hirschsprung's disease

Extraintestinal disease
    Obstruction of central lymphatics
        Hodgkin's disease/lymphoma
        Retroperitoneal fibrosis
        Thoracic duct obstruction
    Raised central venous pressure
        Constrictive pericarditis
        Tricuspid valvular disease
        Superior vena cava obstruction

— Mechanisms often ill understood but loss is associated with
  - Rapid mucosal cell turnover
    - Menetrier's disease,
    - Coeliac disease
    - Ulcerative colitis
  - Lymphatic stasis
    - Intestinal lymphangiectasia
    - Thoracic duct obstruction
  - Venous stasis
    - Malrotation
    - Constrictive pericarditis
    - Table 9.1 is therefore arranged anatomically

Clinical features

— Failure to thrive
— Hypoproteinaemic oedema
— Ascites and pleural effusion (clear or chylous)
— Features of causative disorder
— Hepatomegaly in severe long-standing disease
— Lymphoedema associated with
  - Intestinal lymphangiectasis – localised
  - Obstruction of central lymphatics – localised or generalised

Investigation

— Exclude
  - Cirrhosis
  - Renal protein loss
— Measure faecal alpha-1-antitrypsin excretion as a semi-quantitative measure of protein loss
  - Stool clearance of alpha-1-antitrypsin (faecal concentration × daily stool weight/serum concentration) overcomes need to use radioactive marker
    - Good correlation with ^{51}Cr-labelled albumin excretion
    - 4 day stool collection
    - Normal <13 ml/day
    - Random stool alpha-1-antitrypsin concentration is a good screening test ($n < 3.4$ mg/g dry stool)
— ^{51}Cr-labelled albumin excretion test
  - 925 kBq of ^{51}Cr-labelled albumin or ^{51}CrCl$_3$ given intravenously
  - All stools collected for four days taking meticulous care to avoid urine contamination
  - Greater than 1% excretion in stools is abnormal
  - Greater than 4% is diagnostic
  - Most patients with symptoms have losses of 10 to 25%

— Protein loss is nearly always non-selective
  • Plasma protein electrophoresis reflects differential synthesis rate
  • Albumin and immunoglobulins characteristically grossly reduced
— Lymphopenia is common and sometimes severe if protein loss is from lymphatics

Intestinal lymphangiectasia

—Intestinal lymphangiectasia should be sought in the absence of other obvious cause
— Contrast radiology
  • Often shows characteristic coarse mucosal folds
  • May suggest site for likely positive findings on jejunal biopsy
— Jejunal biopsy (usually from beyond the duodenum)
  • Whitish appearance of some villous tips under dissecting microscope
  • Characteristic club shaped villi on histology and fat in enterocytes and dilated lymphatics in lamina propria on staining
  NB Lesion is very patchy and affects relatively few villi
— Laparotomy
  • Abnormal fat filled lymphatics are seen in the mesentery

Management
— See below

Other diagnoses

— Contrast studies may demonstrate
  • Crohn's disease
  • Malrotation
— Jejunal biopsy may demonstrate
  • Crohn's disease
  • Coeliac disease
  • Eosinophilic gastroenteritis
  • Whipple's disease
  • Venous obstruction (oedema)
  • T-cell deficiency (PAS positive macrophages)
— Barium enema and colonoscopy should be carried out if ulcerative colitis or Crohn's suspected
— Cardiovascular disease is apparent on examination (except constrictive pericarditis)
— Other disorders of lymphatic drainage may require lymphangiography for demonstration

Management

— Correction of the underlying disorder if appropriate
— High protein diet
— In intestinal lymphangiectasia
  - Medium chain triglyceride (MCT) as fat source in diet
    - MCT is absorbed via the portal venous system
    - Diet low in long-chain fat (LCF) reduces lymphatic obstruction
    - Only up to one-third of dietary fat is replaced by MCT is view of possible hepatotoxicity and essential fatty acid deficiency
    - See Appendix B for details of MCT products
  - Low fat diet also effective but
    - Less acceptable to patients
    - May be energy deficient

Prognosis

— There is usually a good response to the above measures in intestinal lymphangiectasia
— Otherwise depends on underlying cause

10 RECURRENT ABDOMINAL PAIN

Definition
— More than three attacks of pain occurring over a period greater than three months

Incidence
— May affect 1 in 10 children and 1 in 4 nine-year-old girls
— Episodes of 'abdominal pain' not strictly defined as above are an almost universal symptom

Aetiology
— Only 5% have an organic illness diagnosed as the cause

ORGANIC

— Always considered in diagnosis
— Clues suggesting organic aetiology
  - Other evidence of organic disease, e.g. growth failure
  - Gross abdominal distension during an episode (NB aerophagy)
  - Site of pain distant from the umbilicus
  - Atypical child (e.g. robust extrovert)
  - No evidence of any family or emotional stress
  - Failure to respond to standard approach (see below)
— Always take careful 'organically oriented' history and do physical examination (see management plan below)
— Obtain longitudinal growth data
— Arrange to see child during an episode
— Perform erect abdominal X-ray during an episode if distension is a feature
— Limited investigations always include urine microbiology, haemoglobin and ESR
— See Table 10.1 listing some important though rare causes of recurrent abdominal pain

Table 10.1 Important organic causes of recurrent abdominal pain as an isolated symptom

Recurrent, subacute intestinal obstruction
Intussusception
Malrotation
Duplication
Volvulus
Internal herniae
Stenosis
Aerophagy
Cholecystitis
Cholelithiasis
Urinary tract
   Infection
   Pelviureteric obstruction
   Stone
Splenic infarction
Ovarian tumours/cysts
Referred spinal pain
Tuberculosis
Crohn's disease
Peptic ulcer
Pancreatitis
Lead poisoning
Porphyria

Peptic ulceration

— Night pain common
— Family history of peptic ulcer common

Gastric ulcer

— Rare in children and rarely causes this syndrome
— Occurs in
  - The neonatal period
  - Acute stress (e.g. burns)
  - With intracranial pathology
  - With salicylates or other drugs
  - Acute gastric erosions of unknown cause

Duodenal ulcer

— Comparatively rare though apparently commoner in children in the USA than in the UK
— Usual presentation is recurrent pain
  - Rarely has typical features as seen in adults
  - May not occur in young children
— Vomiting is commoner presentation than in adults
— Epigastric tenderness usually present
— Evidence of occult blood loss or iron deficiency anaemia
— Diagnosis by contrast radiology should be confirmed endoscopically in view of rarity and importance of diagnosis to the child
— Management conservative in the first instance
  - Antacids
  - H_2 receptor antagonists

— Relapses occur
— If surgery is required operation of choice is probably selective vagotomy and pyloroplasty

Peptic oesophagitis
— Relatively common in children
— Symptoms of regurgitation and/or dysphagia are usually present
— Commonly occurs in children with cerebral palsy

FUNCTIONAL

— Syndrome has a functional basis in 95% of patients
— Apley has suggested a useful schematic representation of psychosomatic disorders on which Figure 10.1 is based
  • The 'normal' response to stress is a period of arousal, anger, sadness, excitement, etc., followed by adjustment and a return to the previous state
  • Failure to make this adjustment and additional factors shown in the figure contribute to the development of psychosomatic symptoms

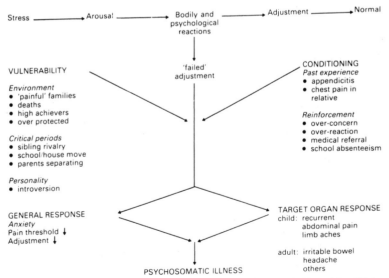

Figure 10.1 The pathophysiology of psychosomatic illness (recurrent pain syndrome) (modified from Apley)

- Children may be vulnerable due to their personality, their environment or both
- Inappropriate responses by parents or professionals may reinforce minor symptoms
- Previous experience may affect the type of symptoms produced (e.g. parent with peptic ulcer)
- The particular type of recurrent pain syndrome appears to be age related. See Figure 10.1, Target organ response
- The general response contributes to the target organ response by an increase in anxiety and decreased adjustment and pain threshold

— Characteristics of the pain
  - Usually periumbilical
  - Often severe but short-lived
  - Site may be determined by previous experience, e.g. appendicectomy
  - Rarely interferes with appetite or voluntary activity
  - May occur at specific times (e.g. on school mornings, at bedtimes)

— Associated symptoms and signs may reinforce 'organic' nature of pain to parents and professionals. They may include:
  - Nausea
  - Lassitude
  - Pallor
  - Abdominal distension
  - Low grade pyrexia
  - Other pains, e.g. headache, limb aches
  - Change in stool habit

Management

Directed towards
  — Optimal therapy for functional disorder
  — Excluding organic cause
    NB Because main emphasis is rightly on a functional disorder organic causes may be missed initially but will be diagnosed when 'functional' management fails or new features appear (e.g. weight loss)

Initial consultation
  — Aims
    - Gain confidence of parents and child
    - Exclude obvious organic pathology
    - Sow the seeds of a possible functional cause
  — Take a full medical history
  — Superficial exploration of likely areas of stress
    - Family stress
    - Move of house or school
    - Death of close family friends, relatives or pets

- Separation experience
- Sibling rivalries
- School friendships/problems
— Assess growth status
— Full physical examination is essential to reassure both doctor and family
— Simple investigations including
  - Urine microbiology
  - The 'necessary' blood test (haemoglobin)
  - An ESR
  - Perhaps stool microscopy and culture if diarrhoea a symptom
— If organic symptoms are prominent
  - Arrange an appropriate investigation during an episode
    - e.g. erect abdomen X-ray if distension is feature
  - Possibly arrange for the child to be seen during an episode
— Successful consultation results in
  - Reassurance that a thorough examination has found nothing serious
  - Hints that there may be a functional cause in many children with this problem

Subsequent consultation
— Review findings and investigations
— Reassure family that there is no serious problem
— Formally discuss the likely functional aetiology, perhaps at parental and child level separately
— It is rarely profitable to attempt identification of the precipitating or maintenance factors responsible
  - Identification is rarely accurate
  - Unnecessary for simple management
— Point out the frequency of the problem in 'normal' children
— Suggest that it commonly occurs in thoughtful, sensitive children
— Review identified conditioning responses in family and discuss ways of reducing them
  - Reassurance in itself may allow this
— Plan measures to increase child's sense of security in the family
  - Often successful is a plan for one or other parent to give child their **undivided** attention for a short period each day to do something of the child's choice
— Review 4–6 weekly on two occasions
— If no response
  - Re-review possible organic causes
  - Consider formal psychiatric referral

Prognosis

— About 80% respond by disappearance or major reduction in symptoms

— Few present later with different psychosomatic disease if
  disorder is explained to child at his or her own level
— In the long term less than 50% will be free of symptoms as adults
  • Commonest symptom is irritable bowel
  • Peptic ulcer is commoner than in the general population
  • Their children are six times as likely to have recurrent
    abdominal pain than the rest of the population

11 ENCOPRESIS, CONSTIPATION AND SOILING

Physiology of defecation

— The lower rectum is normally empty
— Entry of faecal material from above gives the sensation of needing to defecate
— This sensation is lost if rectum is chronically distended
— The gastrocolic reflex makes defecation more likely after a meal

Definitions and descriptions

Encopresis
— Inappropriate passage of a normal stool
— Faeces passed into the pants, on to the floor or behind furniture, etc.
— It is implied that there is normal sensation and control

Constipation
— Difficulty or delay in the passage of stools
— Implies that the lower rectum is usually full rather than empty
— Does not imply that the faecal material is necessarily hard

Soiling
— Inappropriate passage of stool associated with chronic constipation
— Passage of stool is involuntary and usually unsuspected by patient in contrast to encopresis
— Faecal material may be soft or may be brown liquid leaking past hard faecal 'scybala'
  • Often referred to as constipation with overflow or spurious diarrhoea

Neurogenic soiling
— Soiling which occurs due to a neurological abnormality
— Occurs in spina bifida, myelomeningocoele, paraplegia, etc.

Encopresis

— Major emotional or psychological contribution to pathogenesis
— Exclude constipation by abdominal and rectal examination (and plain X-ray abdomen)

- Formal psychosocial assessment aiming to define and describe the psychodynamics
  - What environmental factors present
  - What precipitated symptom
  - What factors are maintaining it
- Therapy may be behavioural, analytical, family oriented or a combination of these approaches
- Laxatives have no place in management

Constipation and soiling

Presentation

- Most children present at around 3 to 4 years with a history of 6 months to 2 years
- Some are reported always to have been constipated
- A few present in infancy with simple constipation unrelieved by standard remedies
- Spurious diarrhoea
  - Constipation with overflow of liquid or semiliquid faeces
  - History confuses physician
  - Repeated courses of antidiarrhoeals exacerbate condition

Aetiology

- 'Idiopathic' is commonest
  - May follow a short period of constipation associated with an acute illness, holiday or move
  - May follow an anal fissure
  - May be the result of inappropriate toilet training
  - May be associated with an unpleasant toilet, e.g. inadequate privacy at school
- Organic causes (Table 11.1)
  - Commonest and most important are:
    - Hirschsprung's disease (see p. 12)
    - Hypothyroidism
    - Intestinal pseudo-obstruction (see p. 16)
    - Multiple endocrine adenoma syndrome
  - Other causes usually have other more obvious symptoms and signs
    - Anal stenosis

History

- Consider an organic cause especially if
  - Onset 'from birth'
  - Severe constipation during first year of life
  - Failure to thrive/short stature
  - Failure to respond to adequate therapy
- Most patients are boys

Table 11.1 Organic causes of constipation

Newborn

Intestinal obstruction
Anal atresia
Hirschsprung's disease
Meconium ileus
Atresias, strictures, etc.

Infant

Hirschsprung's
Partial intestinal obstruction
  Pyloric stenosis
  Strictures, diaphragms, etc.
Anal stricture
Congenital adrenal hyperplasia
Hypothyroidism
Renal tubular acidosis
Diabetes insipidus, etc.

Child

Hypothyroidism
Short segment Hirschsprung's
Anal stricture
Lead poisoning
Hypercalcaemia
Diabetes insipidus
Renal tubular acidosis, etc.

Examination

— Confirmation of the degree of constipation by abdominal and rectal examination is mandatory
  - In an infant, the characteristic features of Hirschsprung's may be noted (see p. 13)
  - Always be alert for hypothyroidism

Investigation

— Exclusion of hypothyroidism by measuring plasma thyroxine is almost routine and reassures family that 'tests' have been done
— Exclusion of Hirschsprung's is a major undertaking
  - Barium enema is inadequate for this purpose
  - Rectal biopsy excludes patients with classical Hirschsprung's
  - Anal pressure studies have been interpreted as showing 'ultra-short segment' disease in some centres
— Examination under anaesthetic and four finger anal dilatation is practised in some centres as an investigation. It is not routine
— Organic causes are more likely in infants

Psychosocial assessment/referral

— In many cases, can be appropriately carried out by paediatrician
— If there is obvious significant family pathology, early referral is preferred by psychologists and psychiatrists and makes management easier

Outpatient management
— Establish working diagnosis
— Inform family that it is 'a common problem'
— Give good prognosis

Explain physiology
— Loss of normal sensation
  • Loss of bowel habit
  • Failure to appreciate when bowels open
  • 'He can't help it now'
  NB Illustration of loss sensation by asking parent if they can feel a ring on the finger is a useful gambit

Explain rationale of therapy
— Need to get and keep rectum empty
— Need for large soft faeces
— Need for regular bowel habit

Achieving empty rectum
— Clinicians vary in their approach and families vary in what therapy is acceptable
— Example
  • Regular suppositories daily (2–10 days) until only a small result (e.g. adult Dulcolax in 4 years plus)
  • Others use one or two outpatient enemas
  • Others prefer no rectal treatment and use laxatives only (e.g. 'Picolax')
  • Some clinicians use no medications

Achieving large soft faeces
— Diet is essential ancillary treatment
  • Good daily intake of high fibre diet, or
  • Normal diet + 2–4 tablespoons of bran on cereal in soup, yogurt, etc.
  • Introduce high fibre cereals and recipes
— Many children also need medication at least initially
  • Use lactulose (Duphalac) 5–15 ml twice daily or docusate sodium (Dioctyl-Medo) 12.5 mg t.d.s.
  • Some use a stimulant such as senna (Senokot 2.5–10 ml b.d.) or bisacodyl (Dulcolax 2.5–5 mg b.d.)

Achieving a regular bowel habit
— Behaviour modification techniques are usually used
— Explain need for **opportunity** for a bowel action at least twice and preferably three times daily after meals
— Time must be allowed by the family for child to sit on the toilet at these times in a relaxed environment for at least five minutes
— A book or tape used only at this time may be a useful incentive
— Explain that a bowel action is not expected on every occasion but the aim is for about once daily
— Star charts are a useful method of record keeping as well as an incentive even in children up to 10 years

— Other reward systems may be appropriate to the individual child
— May need negative reinforcement by child washing soiled underclothes

Star charts

— Give symbols for lowest level of co-operation required, e.g. sitting on the toilet
— For purposes of record keeping chart appropriate bowel actions
— Give main symbol for a clean day
— Give extra symbol for several (e.g. three) clean days
— Allow a tangible reward for a long period (e.g. a week) clean
  • This should be easily and immediately available so that it can be closely linked to success.

Follow up

— Initial frequent follow up is required particularly if the parents have been asked to use suppositories
— Regular follow up at 4–6 week intervals after some success is achieved without reduction of medication, checking diet carefully
— Gradual reduction of medication over several months with maintained or increased fibre intake

Inpatient management

— Rarely required in the first instance
— Management scheme very similar using enemas to speed emptying of rectum
— Careful selection of motivated nurse supervisors
— Continued regular attention during hospital stay with daily inspection of chart by supervising professional (nurse, doctor or psychologist)
— Weekend leave is often a useful manoeuvre to give child and parents sufficient confidence to cope at home

Non-responders

— Careful re-evaluation of possibility of organic disease
— Full and formal psychological assessment

Prognosis

— Long-term prognosis is excellent – very few adults soil!
— Prognosis probably worse in girls
— Short-term results using above scheme are good with approximately 80% success
— Relapse is not uncommon but may be managed along the same lines

Neurogenic soiling

Soiling with physical handicap

— Problems of bowel control are very distressing to intelligent physically handicapped children

- Diet, softening agents, regular opportunities for a bowel action after meals and abdominal compression often result in satisfactory control
- Even if control cannot be achieved chronic constipation should be avoided

Soiling with mental handicap

- Toilet training should be attempted as soon as the child has reached an appropriate developmental stage
  NB This is in social development rather than language or motor
- Behavioural therapy may be instituted from the beginning
- Attempts should be repeated regularly but not continued indefinitely and not repeated too frequently

12 LIVER DISORDERS

NEONATAL UNCONJUGATED JAUNDICE

Physiological

Aetiology
- — Increased bilirubin production
  - Shortened red blood cell survival
  - Increased 'early labelled bilirubin'
- — Reduced bilirubin clearance
  - Patent ductus venosus
  - Reduced bilirubin conjugation
- — Increased small intestinal reabsorption of bilirubin

Variables influencing peak plasma bilirubin concentrations in normal neonates
- — Increased by
  - Delayed cord clamping
  - Breast-feeding
  - Delayed gut transit
  - Oxytocin
  - Hypoxia
  - Hypoglycaemia
  - Dehydration
  - Racial factors (higher in Orientals and Navajo Indians)
- — Decreased by
  - Maternal smoking
  - ?Other drugs (e.g. phenobarbitone)

Pathological

Definition
- — One or more of
  - Clinical jaundice in first 24 h
  - Total bilirubin >220 μmol/l in term infant (>255 μmol/l in pre-term infant)
  - Plasma bilirubin rising at >85 μmol/l/day

- Clinical jaundice in an ill baby
- Persistence of visible jaundice beyond 1 week of age in a term infant (2 weeks in a preterm infant)

Aetiology and management
— See Table 12.1 and Figure 12.1

Table 12.1 Causes of pathological unconjugated neonatal jaundice

Haemolytic
    Blood group incompatibility (Rh, ABO, others)
    Structural erythrocyte defect – hereditary spherocytosis
    Enzymatic erythrocyte defect – G6PD, pyruvate kinase deficiency
    Haemoglobinopathy (rare) – alpha-thalassaemia

Extravascular blood
    Haematoma, bruising, caput, swallowed maternal blood

Bacterial infection ⎱
Metabolic ⎰ also cause cholestasis
    Galactosaemia
Hypothyroidism ⎰

Intestinal obstruction
    Pyloric stenosis, ileal atresia, meconium ileus, Hirschsprung's

Breast milk jaundice

Crigler-Najjar (rare)

Breast milk jaundice
— 'Early' (first week)
- May be a spurious association (more bottle feeding mothers smoke)
- May be due to lower calorie intake or slower gut transit
— 'Late' (after first week)
- Affects 2.5% breast-fed babies
- Associated with elevated lipoprotein lipase and long chain free fatty acids in breast milk

Management
— See Figure 12.1
— Exclude
- Infection
- Hypothyroidism
- Haemolysis
- Cholestasis
- Galactosaemia
— If bilirubin approaches 340 µmol/l, interrupt breast-feeding for 48 h (express milk)
— Resumption of breast-feeding causes a secondary rise which does not reach former peak

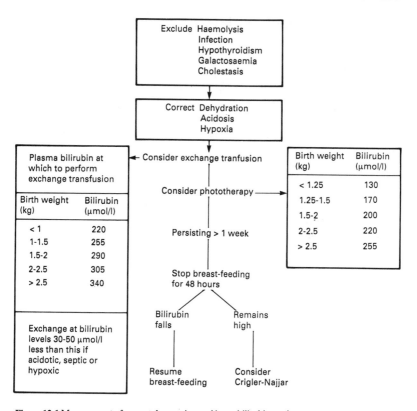

Figure 12.1 Management of neonatal unconjugated hyperbilirubinaemia

---

CONJUGATED HYPERBILIRUBINAEMIA IN INFANCY

— Defined as serum conjugated bilirubin >25 µmol/l
— Always pathological
— Needs urgent investigation
  • To rule out life threatening situations
    – Sepsis (blood and urine culture)
    – Coagulopathy (Clotting studies. Liver disease may present as late onset haemorrhagic disease of the newborn)
    – Galactosaemia (urinary sugars, erythrocyte galactose-1-phosphate, galactokinase, gal-1-P-uridyl transferase)
  • To diagnose or exclude biliary atresia
    – Which requires surgery before 60 days of age

Assessment of cholestatic infant

Clinical examination
- — Syndromes
  - • Alagille's (murmur, facies, retinopathy)
  - • Zellweger (hypotonia, flat facies, flat occiput, high forehead, large fontanelle)
  - • Evidence of chromosomal anomaly, dysmorphic
- — Intrauterine infection (small for dates, purpura, congenital heart disease)
- — Hepatosplenomegaly not useful in discriminating hepatocellular from obstructive causes

Laboratory tests
- — Liver function tests not useful in discrimination
- — See below under Causes for other tests

Determining biliary patency
- — See Figure 12.2

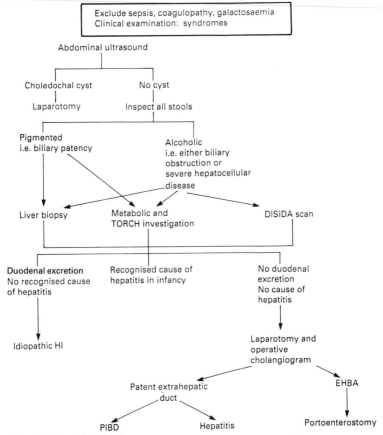

Figure 12.2 Cholestasis in infancy

Causes

— Sepsis
— Obstructive lesions of bile ducts
- ● Biliary atresia
- ● Choledochal cyst
- ● Other anatomical bile duct lesions
— Intrahepatic cholestasis
- ● Neonatal hepatitis (see below)
- ● Biliary hypoplasia
  - – Alagille's syndrome
  - – Non-syndromic

Neonatal hepatitis

— Better called hepatitis of infancy
- ● May occur after 28 days of life

Causes and relevant investigations

— Infective
- ● Hepatitis B
  - – Check maternal HbsAg status
  - – Check infant HBV markers
  - – Manage as in Figure 12.3
- ● CMV
  - – Check for CMV specific IgM
  - – Urine culture

  NB Positive tests first found after 10 days of age likely to be a postnatally acquired infection unless intracranial calcification present
- ● Syphilis
- ● Toxoplasma
— Metabolic
- ● Alpha-1-antitrypsin deficiency
  - – Check Pi phenotype not alpha-1-antitrypsin level
- ● Cystic fibrosis
  - – Plasma immunoreactive trypsin
  - – Stool chymotrypsin
  - – Sweat test
  - – DNA analysis
- ● Galactosaemia
  - – RBC galactose-1-phosphate level and galactose-1-phosphate uridyl transferase activity
- ● Fructose intolerance
  - – Urinary reducing substances present if receiving sucrose
- ● Tyrosinaemia I
  - – Urinary succinyl acetone
  - – Alphafetoprotein

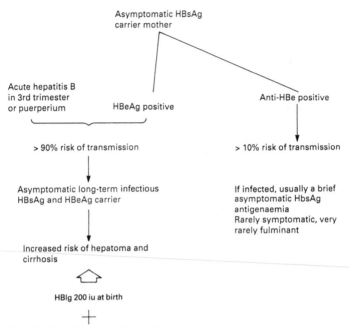

Figure 12.3 Perinatal hepatitis B transmission

- Zellweger syndrome (NB characteristic faeces)
  - Plasma very long chain fatty acids
- Histiocytosis
  - Bone marrow
— Chromosomal
— Endocrine
  - Hypothyroidism/hypopituitarism
— Idiopathic

Extrahepatic biliary atresia

Incidence
— 1:4000 live births
— Causes one-third of infantile cholestasis
— M:F roughly 1:2

Aetiology
— Unknown
— Progressive fibrosing obliteration of extrahepatic and intra-hepatic bile ducts

— Other congenital anomalies in 25%
  - Vascular anomalies
  - Malrotation
  - Polysplenia

Clinical features
— Usually in full-term baby
— Physiological jaundice merges into cholestasis
— Hepatosplenomegaly
— Stools pale from the start in 80–85%
— May present as haemorrhagic disease of the newborn

Diagnosis
— See above under Assessment and Figure 12.1

Operative management
— A small number have a patent biliary system containing proximal common bile duct
  - Anastomose to jejunum in Roux-en-Y
— Remainder
  - Excise extrahepatic biliary system
  - Anastomose intestinal conduit to denuded porta hepatis
    – Portoenterostomy – Kasai procedure

Postoperative problems
— Cholangitis
  - Affects 40–60% in first year postoperatively, less thereafter
  - Adversely affects long-term prognosis in 50% of those involved
    – 5-year survival without cholangitis – 90%
    – 5-year survival with cholangitis – 50%
  - Suspect in any febrile episode post portoenterostomy
    – Blood cultures
    – Blood spectrum IV antibiotics
— Portal hypertension
  - Varices occur in 40–80% of survivors at 5 years
  - Bleeding occurs in 10–20%
  - Injection sclerotherapy preferred first line treatment
— Malnutrition
  - Common
  - High energy diet
  - Fat soluble vitamin supplements
— Cirrhosis

Prognosis after surgery
— Results much worse after late portoenterostomy
  - Surgery before 8 weeks 86% successful
  - Surgery after 8 weeks 36% successful
— Liver transplantation second choice to portoenterostomy
  - Likelihood of success not affected by previous portoenterostomy

- Consider in survivor with
  - Deteriorating liver function
  - Life threatening portal hypertension

Choledochal cyst

— Choledochal cyst is one of a spectrum of anatomical bile duct abnormalities
  - Spontaneous rupture of lower end of duct
  - Stricture
  - Long common channel with pancreatic duct
    - Associated with cholangitis/pancreatitis
— May present after infancy with triad of
  - Pain
  - Mass
  - Jaundice
— Choledochal cysts should be excised
  - Drainage leaves risk of later malignancy

JAUNDICE IN LATER CHILDHOOD

Unconjugated

— Haemolysis most common cause
— Defective conjugation (familial hyperbilirubinaemias; Table 12.2)

Cholestatic

— Plasma unconjugated and conjugated bilirubin raised

Table 12.2 Familial unconjugated hyperbilirubinaemias

| | Gilbert | Crigler–Najjar | |
		Type I	Type II
Age when usually recognised	After puberty	Neonate	First year
Symptoms	Non-specific	Kernicterus	Usually none
Bilirubin in the absence of fasting (mmol/l)	<70	300–850 usually >340	100–800 usually <340
Response to phenobarbitone	Yes	No	Yes
Incidence	5–7%	Rare	Rare
Treatment	None	Phototherapy Transplant	Phenobarbitone

Hepatocellular disease
- — Transaminases elevated
  - • Acute hepatitis syndromes
  - • Chronic hepatitis
  - • Metabolic, e.g. Wilson's
  - • Drug induced, e.g. isoniazid
  - • Decompensated cirrhosis
  - • See below (infective hepatitis)

Dubin–Johnson and Rotor syndromes

- — Rare

Biliary obstruction

- — Alkaline phosphatase and gamma-glutamyl transferase high
- — Congenital
  - • Choledochal cyst
  - • Caroli's disease
  - • Uncorrected biliary atresia
- — Acquired
  - • Calculi
  - • Sludge
  - • Porta hepatis lymphadenopathy
  - • Primary sclerosing cholangitis
  - • Ascending cholangitis
  - • Intrahepatic mass (tumour, abscess, cyst)
  - • Pancreatic fibrosis (cystic fibrosis)

Infective hepatitis

Causes
- — Hepatitis A
- — Hepatitis B
- — Non-A non-B hepatitis, including
  - • Post-transfusion (mainly hepatitis C)
  - • Epidemic water borne ('hepatitis E')
  - • Sporadic
- — Delta hepatitis (hepatitis D)
- — In other viral infections in which other features dominate the clinical picture, e.g.
  - • CMV
  - • EBV
  - • Yellow fever
  - • Adenoviruses
  - • Viral haemorrhagic fevers
  - • Severe varicella zoster

- Measles
- Rubella
— An acute hepatitic illness resembling a viral hepatitis may also be caused by
  - Leptospirosis
  - Malaria
  - Bacteraemia causing cholestasis and/or disseminated intravascular coagulation (DIC)
  - Drugs e.g. isoniazid, cytotoxic agents
  - Budd–Chiari syndrome
  - Liver graft rejection
  - Sickle cell anaemia

Hepatitis A (HA)
— Faecal-oral spread
— Parenteral transmission reported in preterm infants
— Incubation 15–40 days
— Nausea, vomiting, abdominal pain and malaise precede jaundice
— Approximately one-third symptomatic children do not develop jaundice
— Diagnosis by hepatitis A IgM serology
— 70% resolve within 30 days

Variants
— Polyphasic course (second asymptomatic rise in transaminases)
— Cholestasis
— Fulminant hepatic failure
  - Suspect if
    - Unremitting vomiting
    - Child confused or disorientated
    - Prothrombin time prolonged
— Rare associations
  - Henoch–Schönlein purpura
  - Guillain-Barré syndrome
  - Marrow aplasia

Treatment
— None
— Avoid drugs

Prevention
— Gamma-globulin
  - 0.02 ml/kg IM for children travelling to endemic areas for less than 2 months
  - 0.06 ml/kg every 5 months for a prolonged visit (unnecessary if IgG anti-HA present)

Hepatitis B (HB)
Transmission
— Perinatal from
  - HBe antigen (HBeAg) carrier mother
  - Mother with acute, perinatal hepatitis B

— Intrafamilial from mother or siblings
— In developed countries HBV usually spread by deliberate percutaneous puncture
— Use of blood products
  • Factor concentrates in haemophiliacs
  • Thalasssaemia
  • Dialysis
— Tattooing
— Intravenous drug abuse
— Biting and scratching in institutionalised retarded children

Clinical features
— Incubation 3–6 months
— HBV infection may cause acute hepatitis which may be
  • Asymptomatic
  • Symptomatic
  • Severe, or fulminant
— Suspect HBV in acute hepatitis if
  • History of contact
  • Gradual onset
  • Malaise persists after jaundice appears
  • Rash
  • Arthralgia
— May be followed by recovery with anti-HBs or acquisition of the carrier state
— Risk of chronic carrier state increased by
  • Younger age
  • Immunosuppression
  • Asymptomatic infection
  • Down syndrome
  • Chronic renal failure

Diagnosis
— HB surface antigen (HBsAg)
  • Appears in serum 3–6 weeks after infection (2–8 weeks before symptoms)
  • Persists during clinical hepatitis
— In the 'diagnostic window' between HBsAg disappearance and antiHBs antibody appearance, IgM antiHBc (anticore) may be the only marker of HBV

Delta hepatitis (HD, hepatitis D)
— HD is a defective RNA virus requiring presence of HBV
— Co-infection with HBV causes acute hepatitis not distinguishable from HBV alone
  • Variable severity
  • Occasionally fulminant
  • Sometimes bimodal
  • HD disappears with disappearance of HBsAg
— Superinfection of HBsAg carrier causes severe acute hepatitis

- Suspect superinfection if:
  - HBsAg titre low
  - AntiHBe present
  - AntiHBc IgM absent
— High risk of chronic liver disease

Diagnosis
— Delta antibody

Non-A non-B hepatitis (NANB)

Post-transfusion hepatitis (mostly hepatitis C)
— Incidence higher if
  - Paid rather than volunteer blood donors
  - Donor ALT raised
  - If recipient has multiple blood transfusions
  - Risk roughly 3–6/1000 units
— Also transmitted by
  - Coagulation factor concentrates
  - Haemodialysis
  - Organ transplantation
  - IV drug abusers

Hepatitis C
— A cDNA clone isolated from parentally transmitted NANB hepatitis virus
— Probably accounts for most post-transfusion NANB
— Number of other agents involved unknown
— Incubation 7–8 weeks
— Prognosis
  - Cirrhosis in 20% if abnormal LFTs persist >6 months
  - Biopsy may show chronic persistent hepatitis (good prognosis)
  - Biopsy may show chronic active hepatitis (poor prognosis)

Epidemic water-borne hepatitis (hepatitis E)
— Especially in India
— Young adults
— High mortality in pregnancy
— Low risk of chronic liver disease

Sporadic hepatitis
— Usually unknown cause
— Sometimes associated with
  - Needlestick injury
  - Occupational contact
  - Foreign travel

Chronic hepatitis

Investigation
— Liver biopsy is indicated in acute hepatitis which
  - Fails to resolve within 4 weeks and
  - Is not attributable to hepatitis A or B

— Biopsy earlier if
  - Cutaneous stigmata of liver disease
  - Autoantibodies present
  - High immunoglobulins
— Exclude Wilson's disease
— Histology may show chronic persistent hepatitis (CPH) or chronic active hepatitis (CAH)

Chronic persistent hepatitis (CPH)

— Portal triaditis with mild parenchymal damage
— Symptoms mild or absent
— With or without HBV markers
— Good prognosis
— No treatment
— Follow up (occasional evolution to CAH)

Chronic active hepatitis (CAH)

— Hepatitis B, autoimmune, or idiopathic
— Histology shows
  - Portal tract inflammation
  - Piecemeal necrosis
  - Rosetting
  - Septation
  - Bridging necrosis
— Risk of progression to active cirrhosis

Autoimmune chronic active hepatitis

— Hypergammaglobulinaemia ($>20\,g/l$)
— Raised immunoglobulins, particularly IgG ($>16\,g/l$)
— Non-organ specific autoantibodies
  - Smooth muscle antibody (SMA)
  - Liver kidney microsomal antibody (LKMA)
  - Antinuclear antibodies (ANA))
— Liver specific antibodies
  - Anti-liver specific protein (Anti-LSP)
  - Liver membrane antibody (LMA)
— Associations with
  - Other autoimmune diseases
  - Coeliac disease
  - Ulcerative colitis (exclude primary sclerosing cholangitis)

Presentations

— Acute hepatitis which fails to resolve
— May be previous episodes of jaundice
— Insidious onset of systemic symptoms
  - Lethargy
  - Weight loss
  - Abdominal distension
— Cirrhosis on biopsy
— Fulminant hepatic failure

— Asymptomatic abnormality of LFTs on screening affected family members or patients with other autoimmune disease

Management

— Prednisolone 2 mg/kg/day to a maximum of 60 mg/day maintained until ALT < 100 iu
— Prednisolone dose thereafter reduced to lowest dose which maintains biochemical remission
— Azathioprine 0.5–1.5 mg/kg/day has a steroid sparing effect
— Repeat biopsy after 1 year **if**
  • Transaminases normal
  • Autoantibodies negative
  • Serum gammaglobulin not raised
— If no evidence of aggressive inflammation withdraw therapy and follow up closely

HBsAg-positive CAH

— More common than autoimmune in HBV endemic areas
— Tends to evolve to an inactive HBsAg carrier state as viral replication ceases, unless there is delta virus superinfection

Management

— Controversial
  • Traditional view that steroids disadvantageous recently challenged
— Antiviral therapy currently being evaluated

Wilson's disease

Incidence

— 5 per 1 000 000
— Autosomal recessive

Presentation

— Hepatic 40%
— Neurological 35%
— Approximately half present before 15 years of age, most with hepatic disease
  • Insidious onset of lethargy, malaise, anorexia, abdominal pain, with hepatosplenomegaly
  • Acute hepatitis
  • Fulminant hepatic failure with haemolysis
  • Haemolysis alone
  • Portal hypertension
  • Cirrhosis

Investigations

— Slit lamp examination usually fails to show Kaiser–Fleischer rings in first decade
— Serum caeruloplasmin
  • Normal 20–60 mg/dl
  • Wilson's <20 mg/dl

- 5–10% patients with Wilson's disease have values >20 mg/dl if hepatic inflammation present
- 15% heterozygotes have values <20 mg/dl

NB Normal neonates have low values

— Urine copper
  - Normal <70 µg/24 h
  - Wilson's >100 µg/24 h
  - May also be raised in chronic active hepatitis
— After single dose of 20 mg/kg penicillamine
  - Normal urine copper <1 mg/24 h
  - Wilson's >1 mg/24 h
— Serum copper may be normal, low, or high
— Hepatic copper
  - Normal <50 µg/g dry weight
  - Wilson's >250 µg/g dry weight

NB Also elevated in prolonged cholestasis; modest elevation in autoimmune CAH

NB Copper may not be stainable in biopsy sections in first decade, even if concentration elevated

Management

— Copper chelation
  - Penicillamine 35 mg/kg/day + pyridoxine 50 mg/day
— Adverse reactions
  - Rash
  - Fever
  - Lymphadenopathy
  - Lupus-like reaction
  - Severe proteinuria
— May necessitate change to
  - Trientine 400–800 mg t.d.s.
— Zinc sulphate 150 mg t.d.s. after meals, reduces copper absorption and is additive in effect to penicillamine
— Low copper diet unnecessary
— Wilson's disease presenting with fulminant hepatic failure has poor prognosis without transplantation

Reye syndrome

Definition

— An acute encephalopathy accompanied by microvesicular fatty change in the liver
— May be the presenting feature of several inborn metabolic errors (Table 12.3)
— In older child typically biphasic illness
  - Recovery from a prodromal influenza, varicella, respiratory or gastrointestinal infection

Table 12.3 Causes of microvesicular fatty change and encephalopathy

Reye syndrome

Fatty acid oxidation defects
Medium chain acyl dehydrogenase deficiency
Carnitine palmitoyl transferase deficiency
Multiple acyl dehydrogenase deficiencies
    Severe – glutaric aciduria type II
    Mild – methylmalonic aciduria
   Systemic carnitine deficiency (an entity?)
   Hydroxymethylglutaryl coenzyme A lyase deficiency

Urea cycle defects

Toxic
   Jamaican vomiting sickness
   Sodium valproate
   Salicylates

Alpers' disease (progressive neuronal degeneration of childhood with liver disease)

- Followed 1–3 days later by vomiting and change in conscious level
— In infancy, respiratory or gastrointestinal symptoms if present progress to
  - Encephalopathy
  - Tachypnoea
  - Prominent hepatomegaly
— Avoidance of salicylates has caused reduction in Reye syndrome in older children, so infantile presentation now most common
— Diagnosis is probable if in acute encephalopathy if
  - Serum ammonia >100 μmol/l or
  - AAT >100 iu/l or
  - Prothrombin time is >4 s prolonged

Management

— Avoid lumbar puncture
— Plasma or serum glucose, ammonia, prothrombin time, transaminases, urea, electrolytes, osmolality, haemogram and group
— IV 10% glucose 3 ml/kg/h
— Correct coagulopathy
— Reduce ammonia production
  - Neomycin 25 mg/kg 8-hourly orally, unless parenteral, broad spectrum antibiotics are being given
  - Lactulose enema (300 ml syrup, diluted to 1 litre, give 250 ml)
— Assess and monitor coma stage
— Unless coma grade <2 requires
  - Intubation
  - Ventilation
  - Intracranial pressure monitoring
  - Nurse in a 40° head-up position

— Maintain the cerebral perfusion pressure (CPP) between 50 and 90 mmHg (where CPP = intracranial pressure − mean arterial pressure) by
  - Controlled ventilation to maintain Pco_2 3.5–4.0 kPa (25–30 mmHg)
  - Sedation, with extra doses before procedures, avoid opiates
  - Fluid restriction to 30–80 ml/kg/day depending on age
  - Prevention of pyrexia by tepid sponging
— In the presence of spikes or plateaux of raised ICP check
  - Ventilation
  - Head position
  - Neck compression
  - Blood glucose
  - Level of sedation
— If raised intracranial pressure
  - IV mannitol 0.5 g/kg over 20 min
    - Mannitol 0.25 g/kg may be repeated as required
    - Frusemide 1 mg/kg may be additive, providing serum osmolality is <300 mosmol/kg
— Look for signs of seizure activity by fluctuating
  - ICP
  - Heart rate
  - Pupil size
— If present give IV diazepam (1 mg/year + 1 mg) followed by IV phenytoin 10 mg/kg
— Cooling to 31°C by ice packs may reduce cerebral oxygen requirement

LIVER FAILURE

Definitions

— Fulminant hepatic failure
  - Development of hepatic encephalopathy within 8 weeks of the first sign of liver disease
— 'Late onset hepatic failure'
  - Development of hepatic encephalopathy 8–24 weeks from onset of illness
— 'Chronic hepatocellular failure'
  - Persistent or fluctuant jaundice
  - And/or ascites
  - And/or encephalopathy
  - Caused by chronic liver disease

Fulminant hepatic failure (FHF)

In infancy

— May present with
- Coagulopathy
- Obstructive jaundice
- And/or encephalopathy
— Jaundice may initially be absent
— Important neonatal causes
- Galactosaemia
- Fructose intolerance
- Tyrosinaemia

Causes in older child

— Acute hepatitis
- Measure HA IgM antibodies
- Acute hepatitis B rare in childhood
— Superinfection of HBsAg positive carrier with delta virus may cause fulminant hepatitis
- See p. 00
— Other non-A non-B hepatitides are diagnoses of exclusion
— Drugs
- Halothane
- Paracetamol
- Cytotoxic agents
- Pyrrolizidine alkaloids
- Isoniazid
— After cardiac surgery (Fontan procedure for tricuspid atresia)
— Wilson's disease (p. 126)
— Budd–Chiari syndrome
- Gross hepatomegaly
- Ascites
- Ultrasound evidence of hepatic and/or inferior vena caval occlusion

Management

— Support patient until liver function recurs or transplantation performed
— Assess and monitor coma grade
— Avoid
- Sedatives
- Diuretics
- Antiemetics
— Reduce production of nitrogenous toxins in the gut
- Stop protein feeds
- Neomycin 25 mg/kg 8-hourly orally unless parenteral broad spectrum antibiotics used
- Lactulose orally (1 ml/kg) and by enema 300 ml syrup diluted to 1 litre, give 250 ml.

— Prevent hypoglycaemia
  - Oral glucose polymer
  - IV 50% glucose if oral not tolerated
— Monitor electrolytes
  - Hypokalaemia common
— Acid–base balance
  - Respiratory alkalosis in stage 1 coma requires no action
  - Respiratory acidosis (cerebral hypoventilation or respiratory infection) requires intubation and ventilation
  - Metabolic acidosis if severe requires partial correction with bicarbonate
— Correct clotting abnormalities
  - Clotting factor deficiency
  - Disseminated intravascular coagulation
  - Thrombocytopenia
— Measure prothrombin time daily
  - Vitamin K_1 5 mg daily IV
  - Fresh frozen plasma or factor concentrates as necessary
  - Cimetidine to reduce risk of gastric bleeding
— Sepsis
  - Nurse in isolation
  - Blood culture daily
— Broad spectrum antibiotics if
  - Fever
  - Leucocytosis
  - Chest X-ray abnormalities
  - Unexplained deterioration
— Anticipate renal failure
  - Prerenal
  - Functional
  - Acute tubular necrosis
  - Maintain plasma volume
  - May require peritoneal or haemodialysis
— Pancreatitis
  - Ileus
  - Vomiting
  - Monitor serum amylase
— Liver support
  - Exchange transfusion
  - Peritoneal dialysis
  - Plasmaphoresis of unproven value
  - Haemoperfusion improves results in good centres
  - Liver transplant may be precluded by donor availability but good results in adults

Prognosis

— 65–70% mortality in grade 3 coma
— 85–95% mortality in grade 4 coma

— Survival unlikely if
  - Prothrombin time prolonged by >90 s
  - Grade 4 coma lasts >24 h
  - Convulsions or apnoea occur
  - Major complications (renal failure, pancreatitis, sepsis)
— Rising serum alphafetoprotein suggests favourable prognosis

Hepatic encephalopathy

Aetiology

— Four theories
  - Ammonia
  - Synergistic toxins (ammonia, mercaptans, phenols, free fatty acids)
  - False neurotransmitter
  - GABA

Clinical features

— Early features of portosystemic encephalopathy (PSE) often recognised only in retrospect
  - Mood and behaviour changes
  - Disturbance of sleep rhythm
— Intellectual performance deteriorates
  - Handwriting
  - Drawing
  - Distinguishing between objects of similar size and shape
  - Mental arithmetic
— With progression there is
  - Depression
  - Slow responsiveness
  - Confusion
— Asterixis (characteristic flapping tremor of the outstretched hands) is a late, variable feature
— Finally, increasing sleepiness progresses to coma
— EEG is normal in the early stages
  - Becomes abnormal with more advanced PSE
  - Shows slow waves of the delta variety (1.5–3 cps)
  - Initially episodic and frontal
  - Becomes generalised and constant with progression of encephalopathy

Management

— Precipitating factors should be avoided or promptly detected and treated, including
  - All sedatives
  - Excessive use of diuretics in ascites
  - Gastrointestinal bleeding
  - Sepsis (including spontaneous bacterial peritonitis)

— Lactulose is as effective as neomycin though the combination may be synergistic
  - Hydrolysed by colonic bacteria
  - Reduces ammonia reabsorption by lowering colonic pH
  - Speeding colonic evacuation
— High calorie, low protein diet
  - Protein intake of 0.5–1g/kg/day prevents catabolism but will be inadequate for growth
  - Increase as clinically tolerated
— Branched chain amino acids supplements may enable a positive nitrogen balance to be achieved without precipitating encephalopathy (e.g. Generaid)

CIRRHOSIS

Definition
— Diffuse process
  - Characterised by fibrosis
  - Conversion of normal liver architecture into structurally abnormal nodules
  - Continuing ischaemic injury to hepatocytes causes irreversibility

Classification
— Morphological
  - Micronodular or macronodular
  - Active (inflammatory activity present) or inactive
— Aetiological (Table 12.4)
— Functionally, using Child's score (Table 12.5)

Diagnosis
— Easy if liver
  - Hard
  - Enlarged (especially left lobe)
  - Irregular
  NB Liver may be impalpable and abnormally small to percussion
  NB Micronodular cirrhosis cannot be excluded if liver smooth
— Isotope scan shows
  - Decreased uptake
  - Increased uptake over spleen and vertebrae
— Ultrasound shows
  - Abnormal liver texture
  - Features of portal hypertension

Table 12.4 Causes of cirrhosis

Metabolic
    Carbohydrate – galactosaemia, glycogen storage IV
    Amino acid – tyrosinaemia
    Lipid – Niemann–Pick C
    Alpha-1-antitrypsin deficiency
    Copper – Wilson's disease, Indian childhood cirrhosis
    Iron – haemochromatosis, haemosiderosis

Biliary obstruction

Infection
    Hepatitis B (+ delta)
    Hepatitis C
    Non-A non-B hepatitis

Cystic fibrosis

Autoimmune
    Chronic active hepatitis
    Primary sclerosing cholangitis

Toxic
    Chronic veno-occlusive disease

Table 12.5 Child's score for cirrhosis

	Points		
	1	*2*	*3*
Encephalopathy	None	1–2	3–4
Ascites	Absent	Slight	Moderate
Bilirubin (mmol/l)	<30	30–40	>40
Albumin (g/l)	>35	28–35	<28
Prothrombin time (seconds prolonged)	1–4	4–6	>6

Grade A, 5–6 points; B, 7–9 points; C, >10 points.

Ascites

— Contributing factors include
  - Sodium retention (hyperaldosteronism)
  - Portal hypertension (ascites rarely caused by extrahepatic portal hypertension alone)
  - The liver 'drips' lymph, so ascites has a variable protein content
  - Impaired water clearance
  - Renal impairment

Management

— Ascites should be actively treated only if
  - Causing discomfort
  - Respiratory embarrassment
  - Increasing severity

— Sodium restriction
  • No added salt
  • No salt in cooking
  • Avoid sodium-containing drugs
— Water restriction only if
  • Hyponatraemia or
  • Ascites continues to accumulate
— Diuretics
  • Use cautiously
  • Rate of weight loss should not exceed 100 g/24 h in infancy or 300 g/24 h in older children
  • Spironolactone initially 3 mg/kg daily, cautiously increasing until a negative fluid balance is achieved
  • Potassium canrenoate may be given intravenously in the same dose
  • Loop diuretics (frusemide) should not be used alone but may be added to spironolactone if
    – Ascites refractory
    – Hyperkalaemia
    – Metabolic acidosis
— Therapeutic paracenteses in
  • Refractory ascites
  • Withdraw 50 ml/kg/day
— Peritoneovenous (LeVeen) shunt
  • Offers excellent palliation of malignant ascites
  • High complication rate in cirrhotic ascites
— Spontaneous bacterial infection of ascitic fluid
  • Occurs in the absence of localised intra-abdominal sepsis
  • Pathogens include Gram-negative organisms and *Pneumococcus*
  • May present cryptically with otherwise unexplained deterioration in hepatic or renal function, increase in ascites or increase in encephalopathy
  • Diagnosis may be obvious (fever, abdominal pain, and tenderness)
  • Often misdiagnosed
  • Often fatal
  • Diagnostic paracentesis should be performed in these situations or in the newly presenting patient with unexplained ascites
— Cefotaxime IV is an appropriate initial antibiotic whilst awaiting bacterial cultures
— Renal abnormalities (oliguria and uraemia) may result from
  • Prerenal failure
  • Functional renal failure (hepatorenal syndrome)
  • Acute tubular necrosis and other structural renal disorders

Nutrition in cirrhosis

— Malnutrition in cirrhosis may be caused by
  - Anorexia
  - Cholestasis causing malabsorption
  - Therapeutic protein restriction in PSE
  - Geographical association between food shortage and causes of cirrhosis
— The possibility of liver transplantation accentuates the need to keep a potential recipient in as satisfactory a clinical state as possible
— Assessment of nutritional status may be difficult because of fluid overload.
— Patients with established liver disease but without PSE require a standard diet
— If growth is poor extra calories should be provided
  - Fat as tolerated
  - Carbohydrate supplementation as glucose polymers
— Anorexia may be an indication for supplementary enteral feeding with Clinifeed or Fortison (see Appendix B, p. 182) by fine bore nasogastric tube overnight
— Multivitamin preparations should be given
— Fat soluble vitamin status monitored by
  - Serum vitamin A and E
  - Prothrombin time

PORTAL HYPERTENSION

Aetiology
  — See Table 12.6
Presentation
  - Variceal haemorrhage
  - Splenomegaly
  - Hypersplenism
  - Ascites
— If prehepatic
  - Liver small
  - LFTs normal though prothrombin time slightly prolonged
— If intrahepatic
  - Stigmata of causative disease
— If posthepatic
  - Hepatomegaly and ascites prominent
Management
  — Discussed under Management of large bleeds (see p. 90)

Table 12.6 Classification of portal hypertension

Suprahepatic

Constrictive pericarditis
Right ventricular failure
Membranous IVC obstruction
Budd–Chiari syndrome (hepatic vein occlusion) due to:
    Tumour (nephroblastoma)
    Hypercoagulable state
    Polycythaemia
    PNH
    Intrahepatic mass
    Idiopathic

Intrahepatic

Cirrhosis of any cause

Non-cirrhotic

Schistosomiasis
Congenital hepatic fibrosis
Cystic fibrosis
Veno-occlusive disease
Chronic active hepatitis

Prehepatic

Portal vein occlusion
Congenital thrombus
Extrinsic compression
Increased flow
Massive splenomegaly
Splanchnic AV fistula

LIVER TRANSPLANTATION

— Currently two paediatric centres in UK
— Improved results due to
  - Immunosuppression (cyclosporin A)
  - Technical improvements particularly biliary anastomosis
  - Improved donor liver availability and procurement techniques
  - Supportive care

Indications

— Irreversible liver disease with progressive downhill course, e.g.
  - Biliary atresia with unsuccessful Kasai operation
  - Alpha-1-antitrypsin deficiency
  - Wilson's disease
  - Fulminant hepatic failure
— Do not delay until general condition deteriorates

Contraindications
- Absolute
  - Unresectable malignancy
  - Primary disease not helped by liver replacement, e.g. Alpers' syndrome
  - HIV positive
- Relative
  - Portal vein not patent
  - HBeAg positive
  - Hypoxia from pulmonary arteriovenous shunting
  - Intra-abdominal sepsis

Preoperative assessment
- Confirm the diagnosis
- Assess the severity and if possible the rate of progression of the disease
- Assess complications of disease and start additional therapy if possible
- Assess anatomical suitability for transplantation
- Educate the family and child, if old enough, about liver transplantation

Complications
- Infection
  - Bacterial
  - Fungal (usually *Candida*)
  - *Pneumocystis carinii*
  - Viral (CMV, EBV, varicella)
- Rejection
  - Usually in the first three months after transplantation
  - May be acute or chronic and of variable severity
  - Liver biopsy indicated
  - Acute rejection
    - Intravenous methylprednisolone
    - Monoclonal antilymphocytic globulin
  - Chronic rejection
    - Increased doses of oral immunosuppressive therapy
- Vascular thrombosis
- Renal failure
  - Hepatorenal syndrome ('functional renal failure')
  - Postischaemic acute tubular necrosis
  - Severe prerenal uraemia
  - Cyclosporin nephrotoxicity

Results
- 70–80% 1-year survival
- USA results better because retransplantation possible (more donors)

LIVER TUMOURS

— Rare (0.5–2% paediatric malignancies)
— Primary liver tumours outnumbered by secondary involvement from neuroblastoma, Wilms' tumour, lymphoma or leukaemia
— See Table 12.7

Malignant

— Approximately 65% hepatoblastoma
— 25% hepatocellular
— Remainder mesenchymal (Table 12.7)

Table 12.7 Primary liver tumours in childhood

Benign	Malignant
Mesenchymal	Mesenchymal (rare)
Haemangioendothelioma	Undifferentiated sarcoma
Cavernous haemangioma	Embryonal rhabdomyosarcoma
Hamartoma	Mesenchymoma
	Angiosarcoma
Epithelial	Epithelial
Cysts	Hepatoblastoma
Focal nodular hyperplasia	Fetal
Adenoma	Embryonal
	Mixed
	Anaplastic
	Hepatocellular carcinoma
	Fibrolamellar variant

Hepatoblastoma

— Males > females
— Systemic symptoms + hepatomegaly
— High alphafetoprotein
— Rare clinical associations include
  • Precocious puberty
  • Hypercholesterolaemia
  • Hemihypertrophy
  • Beckwith–Wiedemann syndrome (macrosomia, macroglossia)
— Total primary resection offers best chance of survival

Benign

- — Vascular commonest (Table 12.7)
- — Cavernous haemangiomas may present in first 6 months with
  - Cardiac failure
  - Thrombocytopenia
  - Cutaneous haemangiomata
  - Spontaneously regress
  - May require steroids or hepatic artery ligation for intractable cardiac failure

13 NUTRITION

PROTEIN-ENERGY MALNUTRITION

Definition
- Deficiencies of major body nutrients, resulting from a diet inadequate in energy and protein
- Frequently accompanied by micronutrient deficiencies
- Exacerbated by infections (e.g. measles, gastroenteritis)

Prevalence
- 10^8 children less than 4 years old affected in Africa, Asia and Latin America
- Cause of death of up to half of children under 5 years in underdeveloped countries in association with diarrhoea
- In developed countries seen in hospitals, e.g. children and infants with
  - Crohn's disease
  - Protracted diarrhoea
  - Short gut
  - Postoperative abdominal or cardiothoracic surgery
  - Extensive burns/trauma
  - Cystic fibrosis
  - Anorexia nervosa
  - Severe congenital heart disease
  - Advanced cirrhosis
  - Malignancy
  - Cerebral palsy

Classification
- See Table 13.1

Marasmus
- Greek marasmus, wasting
- Associated with urban environment
- Wizened, wasted appearance

Table 13.1 Characteristics of malnutrition

	Weight as % of mean weight for age	Oedema
Underweight child	80–60	No
Marasmus*	Less than 60	No
Kwashiorkor*	80–60	Yes
Marasmic kwashiorkor	Less than 60	Yes

* See text.

— Abdomen scaphoid or distended
— Subnormal weight velocity, followed by subnormal height velocity, then subnormal head growth
— Decreased skin fold thickness
— Irritability or apathy
— Diarrhoea and dehydration
— Hypothermia

Kwashiorkor

— Ga language of Ghana: disease the first child gets when the second is on the way
— Occurs mainly in rural areas in the second year of life
— Failure to thrive
— Oedema
— Muscle wasting
— Angular stomatitis
— Abdominal distension with hepatomegaly
— Skin pigmentation, hyperkeratosis and desquamation, ulceration maximal in napkin area. Healing with depigmentation
— Hair sparse and depigmented with red or grey streaks and loss of curl
— In spite of oedema, disease is preceded by weight loss
— Skinfold thickness may be preserved if calorie intake adequate
— Irritability of apathy and regression
— Tremors
— Diarrhoea
— Hypothermia, bradycardia, hypotension

Pathogenesis

— Inadequate lactation with early weaning predisposes to marasmus, followed by a diet inadequate in energy and protein
— Kwashiorkor may arise when the child is weaned on to a diet of inadequate protein content

NB Aflatoxin theory

— Epidemics may be precipitated by measles, gastroenteritis or malaria

Differential diagnosis
— Other causes of failure to thrive with (see p. 41) or without (see p. 73) diarrhoea
— Other causes of oedema (cardiac, hepatic, renal and gastrointestinal protein loss)

Biochemical features
— Hypoalbuminaemia
— Low plasma urea
— Hypoglycemia
— Hypokalaemia
  - Leads to alkalosis, as H^+ ions are lost in the urine in exchange for conserved K^+
  - Impairs renal concentration of urine
  - May require prolonged K^+ supplementation to correct
— Hypomagnesaemia

Effects of protein-energy malnutrition

— Protein-energy malnutrition may be a severe multisystem disorder, with the following features:
  - Immunodeficiency (frequent infections)
  - Apathy
  - Gastrointestinal dysfunction (see below)
  - Reduced muscle power
  - Respiratory dysfunction
  - Myocardial dysfunction
  - Growth failure

Gastrointestinal effects of protein energy malnutrition

Stomach
— Hypochlorhydria
— Bacterial contamination
Small intestine
— Mucosa varies from normal to subtotal villus atrophy
— Lamina propria infiltration with plasma cells and lymphocytes
— Reduced mucosal disaccharidase activity
  - Lactase most severely affected and slowest to recover after nutritional rehabilitation
— Small bowel contamination
Colon
— Mucosal atrophy
— Plasma cell infiltration of the lamina propria
Pancreas
— Decreased output of amylase, lipase and trypsin

Liver
- Periportal fatty infiltration
- Due to increased fat mobilisation from adipose tissue and decreased synthesis of beta-lipoproteins which normally transport triglycerides from the liver

Management
- See p. 167

VITAMIN DEFICIENCIES

- Organic food substances
- Required in small amounts (mg/day or less)
- Essential for normal metabolism
- Not synthesised in the body

Water-soluble vitamins

- Water-soluble vitamins are essential coenzymes

Vitamin C (L-ascorbic acid)

Functions
- Maintaining intracellular redox potential (reducing agent)
- Hydroxylation of proline and lysine (important in collagen synthesis)
- Tyrosine oxidation
- Adrenal gland function
- Iron absorption

Important sources
- Citrus fruits
- Green vegetables
- Daily requirement 20–30 mg

Deficiency = scurvy
- Rare because ascorbic acid is found in most fresh foods
- May occur in children in institutions

Pathology
- Defective synthesis of the collagen matrix of bone, dentine and cartilage
- Capillary haemorrhages are due to defective basement membrane lining the capillaries, and intracellular substance joining endothelial cells together

Clinical features
- Swollen, bleeding gums
- Bleeding around hair follicles (perifollicular haemorrhages) and petechiae

— Irritability
— 'Pseudoparalysis' due to painful limbs

Radiological signs

— Subperiosteal haematoma calcification
— 'Ground glass' appearance of metaphysis due to atrophy of bone trabeculae
— Epiphysis surrounded by dense rim of cortical bone: 'smoke-ring' epiphysis

Plasma concentrations

— Plasma concentrations below 1 mg/l (5.7 μmol/l) or white blood cell levels below 70 mg/l (400 μmol/l) indicate a high risk

Treatment

— Ascorbic acid 500 mg daily orally for 1 week
— Parenteral dosing leads to massive urinary losses of ascorbic acid
— Treatment should be given without delay as sudden death may occur
— Correction of dietary practices leading to scurvy
— Remodelling of skeletal changes may take months; the other manifestations resolve rapidly

Prevention

— Provision of fresh citrus fruit juice for infants

Vitamin B$_1$ (thiamin)

Function

— Coenzyme in tricarboxylic acid cycle and hexose monophosphate pathway, as thiamin pyrophosphate

Important sources

— Nuts, peas, beans, pulses, brewer's yeast

Deficiency = beriberi

— Malay: beri = weak
— Can occur when intake of thiamin less than 0.4 mg/1000 cal (96 μg/MJ)
— Infantile beriberi may occur in breast-fed infants of mothers existing on a diet of polished rice which contains 0.15 mg/1000 cal
— Cases are found in India and the Far East

Classification

— Acute high output cardiac failure
  • Death may occur suddenly due to
    – Peripheral vasodilatation
    – Lactic and pyruvic acidosis
    – Inadequate utilisation of pyruvate in tricarboxylic acid cycle
— Aphonic
  • Coughing, choking and aphonia, due to laryngeal oedema
— Pseudomeningeal
  • Drowsiness, meningism
  • Older children may develop the sensory and motor neuropathy of so-called dry beriberi

Diagnosis
- Transketolase activity measured in presence and absence of thiamin pyrophosphate
- Increase in activity of more than 25% indicates deficiency

Treatment
- 50–100 mg thiamin hydrochloride IV or IM immediately diagnosis is suspected, followed by 5–10 mg/day for 1 week
- Response is seen within hours
- If breast-fed the infant's mother should also be treated

Prevention
- Diversification of diet
- Enrichment of rice with thiamin

Nicotinic acid (niacin)

Functions
- Exists in the body as nicotinamide, a constituent of coenzymes NAD^+ and $NADP^+$
- NAD^+ and $NADP^+$ required for many redox reactions
  - Including those of glycolysis, electron transfer, pentose and fatty acid metabolism

Important sources
- Nicotinic aid can be synthesised from tryptophan
- Meat, fish, wholemeal cereals and pulses are richest source of nicotinic acid

Deficiency = pellagra
- Italian: pelle = skin, agra = rough
- Endemic in parts of southern Africa, due to maize diet
  - Low in tryptophan
  - Nicotinic acid in maize has poor bioavailabity
- Deficiency of vitamin B6 (pyridoxine), an essential cofactor in nicotinic acid synthesis from tryptophan, may also lead to pellagra

Clinical features
- Skin
  - Photosensitive dermatitis
  - Progresses to scaling and increased pigmentation
- Gastrointestinal tract
  - Angular stomatitis
  - Cheilosis
  - Diarrhoea
- CNS
  - Depression
  - Delerium
  - Dementia
  - Peripheral neuropathy

Diagnosis
- Typical skin lesions

— Low plasma tryptophan
— Low N-1-methyl nicotinamide and pyridone derivative in urine

Prognosis

— Skin lesions deteriorate in summer
— Mental changes may be permanent

Treatment

— Oral nicotinamide (100 mg 4-hourly)
— Addition of protein to diet

Prevention

— High tryptophan strains of maize (opaque-2)
— Fortification of diet with nicotinamide

Vitamin B₂ (riboflavin)

Deficiency

— May occur if intake >130 µg/MJ (0.55 mg/1000 cal)
— Angular stomatitis and cheilosis
— Magenta coloured tongue
— Nasolabial seborrhoea

Diagnosis

— In riboflavin deficiency erythrocyte glutathione reductase activity increases by 30% or more after addition of FAD in vitro

Treatment

— Riboflavin 20 mg/day to initiate treatment

Prevention

— Consumption of legumes, pulses and animal products

Vitamin B₆ (pyridoxine)

Functions

— Coenzyme for over 60 different enzymes, mainly involved in amino acid metabolism

Important sources

— Liver, whole grain cereals, peanuts and bananas
— Widely distributed in food, hence deficiency rare

Deficiency (see also Nicotinic acid p. 146)

— Apart from malnutrition and malabsorption, certain drugs antagonise pyridoxine
  • Notably isoniazid, hydrallazine, penicillamine and oestrogens
— Convulsions may result from deficiency of gamma-aminobutyric acid, an inhibitory CNS neurotransmitter the synthesis of which is pyridoxine dependent
— Peripheral neuropathy
— Depression

Diagnosis

— Serum pyridoxal 5'-phosphate less than 25 µg/l
— Increase in red cell aspartate and alanine aminotransferases in presence of pyridoxal 5'-phosphate *in vitro*
  • By more than 100 and 25% respectively

Treatment
— Pyridoxine 10 mg/day

Folic acid (folate, folacin, pteroylglutamic acid)
Functions
— Transfer of CH_3 into deoxyuridylic acid to form thymidylic acid: constituent of DNA
— Vitamin B_{12} required for conversion of the inactive CH_3 tetrahydrofolic acid to tetrahydrofolic acid
  • Hence interdependence of B_{12} and folic acid in DNA synthesis

Important sources
— Liver, kidney, broccoli, spinach, cabbage
— Preparation of food can cause severe losses

Deficiency
— May arise from
  • Dietary deficiency
  • Increased requirement (e.g. haemolytic anaemia)
  • Malabsorption
  • Use of folate antagonists
    – Including phenytoin, methotrexate, trimethoprim and pyrimethamine
— Causes megaloblastic anaemia

Diagnosis
— Lowered red cell folate (normal range 160–640 µg/l)
  • Is a better indicator of deficiency than plasma folate (6–12 µg/l)
  • Plasma reflects recent dietary intake
— Macrocytic anaemia with hypersegmented neutrophils and megaloblastic bone marrow
— Thrombocytopenia in severe deficiency

Treatment
— Folic acid 1–5 mg/day
— IV folinic acid 3 mg for methotrexate toxicity

Vitamin B_{12} (cobalamin)

Functions
— DNA synthesis (see folic acid)
— Maintenance of myelin via role in propionyl CoA catabolism

Important sources
— All animal-derived foodstuffs: vitamin B_{12} absent from vegetable foodstuffs

Deficiency
— Causes of B_{12} deficiency in childhood are shown in Table 13.2
  • All are rare
— Sufficient stores for several years normally present in liver
— Symptoms and signs: anaemia, yellow tint to skin, glossitis, paraesthesia, ataxia, dementia

Table 13.2 Causes of vitamin B_{12} deficiency in childhood

Cause	Example
Inadequate intake	Vegan diet
Inadequate absorption	Intrinsic factor deficiency
	Production of biologically inactive intrinsic factor
	Intraluminal binding in small bowel overgrowth
	Ileal disease: Crohn's, ileal resection
Inadequate distribution	Plasma B_{12} transport protein (transcobalamin II) deficiency

Diagnosis
- Plasma normal range 150–1000 ng/l
- Deficiency associated with megaloblastic anaemia, hypersegmented polymorphs and thrombocytopenia
- Schilling test (see p. 179)

Treatment
- 1000 μg B_{12} twice weekly until haemoglobin normal then 6-weekly IM
- If malabsorption, rather than intrinsic factor deficiency is responsible, large oral doses (25–50 μg) may be tried

Pantothenic acid
- Spontaneous deficiency in man not reported

Biotin
- Deficiency seen only after massive consumption of raw egg (contains binding protein)

Fat-soluble vitamins

- Are not coenzymes
- Probably function by altering protein conformation
- Vitamin toxicity confined to fat-soluble vitamins

Vitamin A (retinol)

Functions
- Essential component of retinal pigment rhodopsin (visual purple)
- Deficiency leads to squamous metaplasia of epithelial surfaces

Important sources
- Animal: liver, milk, butter, cheese, eggs
- Plant: the pigment carotene is a dimer of vitamin A
- Destroyed by light

Deficiency
- May occur when diet lacks dairy produce, fresh vegetables and fruit
- Xerophthalmia
  - Conjunctival xerosis – dry wrinkled conjunctiva with white foamy plaque (Bitot spot)

- Corneal xerosis – clouding of cornea due to keratinisation
- Keratomalacia – necrosis of cornea
— Follicular hyperkeratosis: blocking of sebaceous glands with keratin plugs (also may be seen in malnutrition and essential fatty acid deficiency)

Diagnosis
— Confirmed by vitamin A level of less than $200\,\mu g/l$ and carotenoids less than $500\,\mu g/l$

Treatment
— 300 mg retinol (1 dose orally, 1 IM) for 3 days, then 9 mg/day orally for 2 weeks)

Prevention
— Encouraging intake of green, leafy vegetables and yellow or orange fruit
— 60 mg retinol every 6 months in endemic areas

Vitamin D (cholecalciferol)
— Cholecalciferol (vitamin D_3) is produced from 7-dehydro-cholesterol (from animal fat) by UV light
— Ergocalciferol (vitamin D_2) is produced from ergosterol (from yeast) by UV light

Functions
— Vitamin D of dietary or cutaneous origin hydroxylated
- In the liver to 25-OH vitamin D_1
- Then in the kidney to $+$ 1,25-$(OH)_2$ vitamin D (ten times more active than vitamin D)
— Renal synthesis of 1,25-$(OH)_2$ vitamin D stimulated by parathormone
— 1,25-$(OH)_2$ cholecalciferol
- Induces synthesis of Ca^{2+} binding protein in jejunal enterocytes which promotes Ca^{2+} absorption
- Mobilises Ca^{2+} from bone in presence of parathormone
- Stimulates ileal phosphate absorption

Important sources
— Ergocalciferol from skin most important source
— Oily fish chief dietary source, with fortified margarine
— Dairy products relatively poor source as is breast milk

Deficiency = rickets
— Anglo-Saxon: wrikken = twist
— Defective calcification of metaphyseal cartilage in growing children due to vitamin D deficiency
— Vitamin D deficiency in adults is called osteomalacia
— Common in cities in UK, especially in Asian children
— Ca^{2+} and phosphate normal in mild cases
— In severe cases, serum Ca^{2+} falls, as intestinal absorption decreases
- Parathormone production increases, causing hypophos-phataemia due to increased urinary phosphate excretion

— Alkaline phosphatase activity elevated from osteoblasts in metaphyseal uncalcified ('osteoid') tissue
— Skeletal lesions include
  • Craniotabes (softened areas of skull bones, which can be indented)
  • Epiphyseal swelling (most noticeable distal radii)
  • Enlarged costochondral junctions ('rickety rosary')
  • Delayed fontanelle closure
  • 'Bossing' frontal and parietal bones
  • Pectus carinatum ('pigeon chest')
  • Harrison's sulci (depression of rib cage at site of insertion of diaphragm)
  • Genu valgum, tibial bowing
  • Ultimate growth retardation
  • Delayed dentition
— Other features which may occur include irritability, hypotonia and respiratory failure, tetany, laryngospasm, convulsions, aminoaciduria

Diagnosis

— By raised alkaline phosphatase for age, low phosphate and/or Ca^{2+}
— Widening of the metaphyseal plate, and concavity of the ends of the diaphysis (shafts of bone)

Treatment

— Vitamin D 25–125 µg/day (1000–5000 iu/day)
— If compliance is a problem, a single dose of 7.5 mg (300 000 iu) can be given
— Continue until alkaline phosphatase normal, then give prophylactic dose (10 µg/day)
— Ensure 500 ml/day milk to supply Ca^{2+}
— Encourage greater sunlight exposure
— Extensive remodelling of deformed bones occurs, but orthopaedic surgery required for the severest cases

Prevention

— Unless child is receiving a vitamin D fortified milk, 10 µg/day should be administered until 1 year
— Preterm babies especially at risk, because of poor hepatic stores and rapid growth
— Anticonvulsants induce hepatic enzymes which accelerate vitamin D breakdown: epileptic children require prophylaxis

Toxicity

— Excess vitamin D intake causes hypercalcaemia
  • Vomiting, constipation, polyuria, irritability, drowsiness, metastatic calcification, especially blood vessels and kidneys

Vitamin E (tocopherol)
Functions

— Thought to act as a biological reducing agent, preventing damage to cell membranes by O_2

Important sources
— Vegetable oils richest source: eggs, butter, wholemeal cereals moderately rich

Deficiency
— May cause haemolysis in preterm infants and in patients with steatorrhoea
— Neuroretinal complications of abetalipoproteinaemia have been attributed to deficiency
— Presumed in patients with cystic fibrosis

Diagnosis
— RBC susceptible to haemolysis by hydrogen peroxide (30–100% haemolysed)
— Serum vitamin E less than 5 mg/l (less than 1 µg/mg plasma lipid or less than 11 µmol/l)

Treatment
— Tocopherol acetate, 10 mg/kg/24 h in steatorrhoea, 100 mg/kg/24 h in abetalipoproteinaemia

Vitamin K (phytomenadione)

Function
— Cofactor for hepatic synthesis of clotting factors II, VII, IX and X

Important sources
— Green leafy vegetables (vitamin K_1)
— Synthesis by gut flora (vitamin K_2)

Deficiency in newborn = haemorrhagic disease
— May occur after broad spectrum antibiotics
— Preterm infants fed breast milk especially at risk (haemorrhagic disease of the newborn)
— Prothrombin time (and clotting time) prolonged; other clotting tests normal
NB Prolonged prothrombin time may also occur in liver disease, without vitamin K deficiency
NB Accompanied by thrombocytopenia and prolonged partial thromboplastin time suggests disseminated intravascular coagulation

Treatment
— Vitamin K_1 5 mg as required (1 mg in the newborn)
— Larger doses may induce haemolysis, especially in infants with G6PD deficiency

Prevention
— All breast-fed infants should receive prophylaxis
— Most neonatal units now give prophylactic vitamin K to all newborns
  • Some give only to selected 'at risk' newborns
— 1 mg for term infants
— 0.5 mg for preterm
— Usually IM but oral may be adequate in repeated doses

PARENTERAL NUTRITION

Indications
— See Table 13.3

Table 13.3 Indications for parenteral nutrition in paediatric practice

Protracted diarrhoea of infancy
Major alimentary surgery in newborns
Necrotising enterocolitis
Intensive care of low birthweight infants
Inflammatory bowel disease
Severe trauma
Extensive burns
Acute renal failure

— Consider early in:
- Preterm infants
- Severe catabolic states

NB Without food:
- Adult can survive 3 months
- Full-term infant 1 month
- Preterm infant 12 days

Nutrient solutions
— See Table 13.4 and in Tables 13.12 and 13.16

Table 13.4 Composition of macronutrient parenteral nutrition solutions (per litre)

Solution	kcal (MJ)	Amino acids (g)	Fat (g)	Glucose (g)	Na^+ (mmol)	K^+ (mmol)	Ca^{2+} (mmol)	Mg^{2+} (mmol)	Pi (mmol)
Vamin glucose	650* (2.7)	70†	–	100	50	20	2.5	1.5	–
10% glucose	400 (1.7)	–	–	100	–	–	–	–	–
10% Intralipid	1100 (4.6)	–	100	–	–	–	–	–	15
20% Intralipid	2000 (8.4)	–	200	–	–	–	–	–	15

* 400 kcal (1.7 MJ) per litre from 10% glucose.
† 70 g of amino acids are equivalent to 60 g protein.

Amino acids
— Vamin glucose (Kabi Vitrum)
- L-amino acid solution
- Balanced mixture of all essential and non-essential amino acids

- Low solubility of cysteine/cystine requires low pH (5.2)
- Contains 10% glucose
- Osmolality 1100 mmol/kg
— Vamin infant (Kabi Vitrum)
  - Amino acid composition designed specifically for the newborn
  - Recommended amino acid source for patients under 6 months

Carbohydrate
— 10–30% solutions of dextrose
— 5% is isotonic with plasma
— 10–15% is maximum usable in peripheral vein
— 20% usual maximum with unrestricted volume
— 30% in situations requiring fluid restriction

Lipid
— Intralipid 10 or 20% (Kabi Vitrum)
  - Fractionated soy bean oil
— Provides
    – Essential fatty acids
    – Lecithin
    – Phosphate (from egg phospholipid)
    – Vitamin E
  - 85% of fat is unsaturated and polyunsaturated triglyceride
  - 20% solution usually used as results in less hypercholesterolaemia

Electrolytes, trace elements and vitamins
— Additional Na^+ and K^+ to that provided by Vamin glucose are necessary to achieve amounts of Tables 13.12 and 13.16
— In infants, additional Mg^{2+}, Ca^{2+} and trace elements are provided by Ped-el (Kabi Vitrum) (Table 13.5)
  - 4 ml/kg/day provides probable oral requirements for healthy infants
  - May be insufficient in disease states
— In children over 10 kg Addamel (Kabi Vitrum) provides Mg^{2+}, some Ca^{2+} and trace elements but no P (Table 13.5)

Table 13.5 Composition of Ped-el and Addamel

Constituent	Ped-el (per 4 ml)	Addamel (per 0.2 ml)
	(amount administered per kg/day)	
Ca^{2+} (mmol)	0.6	0.1
Mg^{2+} (mmol)	0.1	0.03
Fe^{3+} (µmol)	2.0	1.0
Zn^{2+} (µmol)	0.6	0.4
Cu^{2+} (µmol)	0.3	0.1
Mn^{2+} (µmol)	1.0	0.8
F^- (µmol)	3.0	1.0
I^- (µmol)	0.04	0.02
P (mmol)	0.3	–

— Water-soluble vitamins provided by Solivito (Kabi Vitrum)
  - 1 vial dissolved in 5 ml 10% dextrose. 0.5 ml/kg/day (max 5 ml) is added to Vamin glucose solution or Intralipid
    – Gives amounts in Table 13.6
— Fat-soluble vitamins provided by Vitlipid Infant (Kabi Vitrum)
  - 1 ml/kg/day (max 4 ml) gives amount in Table 13.7

NB Intralipid contains 30 iu vitamin E per litre

Table 13.6 Composition of Solivito

Constituent	Amount administered per kg per day (see text)
Vitamin B$_1$ (thiamine) (mg)	0.12
Vitamin B$_2$ (riboflavin) (mg)	0.18
Nicotinamide (mg)	1.0
Vitamin B$_6$ (pyridoxine) (mg)	0.2
Pantothenic acid (mg)	1.0
Biotin (mg)	0.03
Folic acid (mg)	0.02
Vitamin B$_{12}$ (cyanocobalamin) (µg)	0.02
Vitamin C (ascorbic acid) (mg)	3.0

Table 13.7 Composition of Vitlipid Infant

Constituent	Amount administered per kg per day (see text)
Vitamin A (retinol) (µg) (iu)	100 (333)
Vitamin D$_2$ (calciferol) (µg) (iu)	2.5 (100)
Vitamin K$_1$ (phytomenadione) (µg)	50

Pharmacy-based regimen

— See Tables 13.8–13.12
— Applicable where solutions and additives can be prepared under aseptic conditions (e.g. in a laminar flow cabinet)
— Requirements of fluid, amino acids, carbohydrate, Na$^+$, K$^+$ and Ped-el are prescribed by ward staff
  - Made up in single solution in aseptic conditions
  - An additional amount of fluid and constituents is made up to allow for wastage, filling of drip sets, etc.
  - Solution is then administered over 24 h
— Intralipid and vitamin requirements are calculated to ensure that required amounts of vitamins are given in the day's volume of Intralipid

Table 13.8 Neonates Parenteral Nutrition Regimens 1–6. All amounts are per kg bodyweight/24 h

	Regimen number					
	1	2	3	4	5	6
Amino acid (g)	0.5	0.8	1.0	1.5	2.0	2.5
Carbohydrate (g)	8	10	10	12	12	14
Fat (g)	1	1	2	2	3	3.5
Sodium (mmol)	3	3	3	3	3	3
Potassium (mmol)	2.5	2.5	2.5	2.5	2.5	2.5
Calcium* (mmol)	0.6	0.6	0.6	0.6	0.6	0.6
Magnesium* (mmol)	0.1	0.1	0.1	0.1	0.1	0.1
Phosphate† (mmol)	0.3	0.3	0.3	0.3	0.3	0.3
Solivito N‡ (ml)	1	1	1	1	1	1
Vitlipid N Infant‡ (ml)	1	1	1	1	1	1
Ped-el‡ (ml)	2	2	3	3	3	4

* From Ped-el.
† Only the phosphate content of the Ped-el is included. This should be increased to 0.7 mmol/kg total, using Addiphos if the patient is preterm. The sodium and potassium content of the Addiphos should be included in calculations.
‡ For full prescribing information see appropriate data sheet.

Table 13.9 Babies over 1 month old but under 10 kg bodyweight regimens 7–11. See Table 13.12 for recipe. Regimens 7–10 are used for the first 4 days of parenteral nutrition, regimen 11 is used for day 5 and beyond. All amounts are per kg bodyweight/24 h

	Regimen number				
	7	8	9	10	11
Amino acid (g)	0.5	1.0	1.5	2.0	2.5
Carbohydrate (g)	8	10	12	13	14
Fat (g)	1	1	2	2	3
Sodium (mmol)	3	3	3	3	3
Potassium (mmol)	2.5	2.5	2.5	2.5	2.5
Calcium* (mmol)	0.6	0.6	0.6	0.6	0.6
Magnesium* (mmol)	0.1	0.1	0.1	0.1	0.1
Phosphate† (mmol)	0.3	0.3	0.3	0.3	0.3
Solivito N‡ (ml)	1	1	1	1	1
Vitlipid N Infant‡ (ml)	1	1	1	1	1
Ped-el‡ (ml)	4	4	4	4	4

* From Ped-el.
† Only the phosphate content of the Ped-el is included. This should be increased to 0.7 mmol/kg total, using Addiphos if the patient is preterm. The sodium and potassium content of the Addiphos should be included in calculations.
‡ For full prescribing information see appropriate data sheet.

- Intralipid and vitamin solution infused over 20 h from 10.00 a.m.
- Infusion is stopped at 6.00 a.m. to allow an estimate of fat clearance from serum when daily blood samples are taken
- Lipaemic serum damages blood gas measuring membranes and may give falsely low plasma Na^+ and K^+ results

Table 13.10 Children over 10 kg but under 30 kg bodyweight Regimens 12–13. See Table 13.12 for recipe. Regimen 12 is used for the first two days, regimen 13 subsequently. All amounts given per kg bodyweight/24 h

	Regimen number	
	12	13
Amino acid (g)	1	2
Carbohydrate (g)	4.5	7.5
Fat (g)	1.5	2
Sodium (mmol)	3	3
Potassium (mmol)	2.5	2.5
Calcium* (mmol)	0.1	0.2
Magnesium* (mmol)	0.06	0.07
Phosphate† (mmol)	0	0
Solivito N‡ (ml)	1	1
Vitlipid N Infant‡ (ml)	1	1
Addamel‡ (ml)	0.2	0.2

* From Ped-el.

† Addamel contains no phosphate, but the phosphate content of the Intralipid is assumed to be bioavailable. However, phosphate should be monitored in those patients on long-term feeding, particularly where growth has been retarded prior to nutritional care.

‡ For full prescribing information see appropriate data sheet.

Table 13.11 Children over 30 kg bodyweight Regimens 14–15. See Table 13.12 for recipe. Regimen 14 is used for the first 2 days, Regimen 15 subsequently. All amounts given per kg bodyweight/24 h

	Regimen number	
	14	15
Amino acid (g)	1	1.5
Carbohydrate (g)	2	5
Fat (g)	1	2
Sodium (mmol)	3	3
Potassium (mmol)	2.5	2.5
Calcium* (mmol)	0.1	0.2
Magnesium* (mmol)	0.06	0.06
Phosphate† (mmol)	0	0
Solivito N‡ (ml)	1	1
Vitlipid N‡§ (ml)	1	1
Addamel‡ (ml)	0.2	0.2

* Derived from Addamel + Vamin 9 Glucose only.

† Addamel contains no phosphate, but the phosphate content of the Intralipid is assumed to be bioavailable. However, phosphate should be monitored in those patients on long-term feeding, particularly where growth has been retarded prior to nutritional care.

‡ For full prescribing information see appropriate data sheet.

§ Vitlipid N Infant up to 10 years of age. Vitlipid N Adult subsequently.

Table 13.12 System for parenteral nutrition using commercially available products
All values are given per kg bodyweight/24 h

Patient group	Day of PN	Age (days)	Fluid (ml)	Vamin infant (ml)	Dextrose 5% (ml)	Dextrose 20% (ml)	Intralipid 10% (ml)	Additional Sodium (mmol)	Additional Potassium (mmol)
Neonates	1	3	90	8	42	30	10	3	2.5
including	1	4–5	120	8	82	20	10	3	2.5
low birth	1	6+	150	8	122	10	10	3	2.5
weight	2	4–5	120	12	63	35	10	3	2.5
	2	6+	150	12	103	25	10	3	2.5
	3	5	120	16	94	40	20	3	2.5
	3	6+	150	16	84	30	20	3	2.5
	4	6+	150	24	61	45	20	3	2.5
	5	6+	150	32	38	50	30*	3	2.5
	6	6+	150	40	10	65	35*	3	2.5
Infants	1		150	8	122	10	10	3	2.5
>1 month	2		150	16	99	25	10	3	2.5
<10 kg	3		150	24	61	45	20	3	2.5
	4		150	32	28	60	20	3	2.5
	5		150	40	5	75	30	3	2.5
10–30 kg	1		60	14†	16	15	15	2	2
	3		90	28†	20	20	30	1	1.5
>30 kg	1		36	14†	12	–	10	2	2
	3		60	20†	–	20	20	1	1.5

* For pre-term, reduce to 20 ml/kg only and make up volume with 5% dextrose.
† Vamin 9 Glucose.

Note: Vitamins to be included as in text. Additional phosphate as in Tables 13.8 and 13.9 above.
Trace Elements: If weight <10 kg, add Ped-el 4 ml/kg/day
    If weight >10 kg, add Addamel 0.2 ml/kg/day

- Daily infusion volume must be reduced if serum lipaemic
- Visual evidence is only crude test of lipid clearance
- Weekly triglyceride is a necessary precaution, particularly in newborns

Ward-based regimen

— See Tables 13.13–13.16 for details
— Vamin Dextrose and dextrose solutions are not mixed but given via a double giving set
— NaCl and KCl are added to dextrose solution
— Ped-el is added to Vamin-Dextrose (some Vamin may need to be removed from bottle to allow addition)
— Solivito and Vitlipid Infant are added to Intralipid as indicated in Tables 13.13–13.15

Access to circulation

— Peripheral drips are preferable to central cannulae in the short term because of reduced risk of infection
  - Problems may occur with extravasation and sloughing of skin

Table 13.13 Ward-based parenteral nutrition regimen for children under 10 kg

Infusion fluid		Infusion rate (ml/kg/h)	Duration (h/24 h)
Day 1			
Intralipid 10%		0.5	20 (stop at 0600)
To each 100 ml add	Solivito 5 ml		
	Vitlipid Infant 10 ml		
	(to maximum of 4 ml/day)		
Vamin Dextrose		2.0	8
To each 100 ml add	25 ml Ped-el		
Dextrose 5%		8.0	16
To each 100 ml add	9 mmol NaCl		
	9 mmol KCl		
Infuse Vamin Dextrose for 1 h, then dextrose 5% for 2 h			
Days 2–5			
Intralipid 10%		1.0	20 (stop at 0600)
To each 100 ml add	Solivito 2.5 ml		
	(to maximum of 4 ml/day)		
Vamin Dextrose		3.0	8
To each 100 ml add	17 ml Ped-el		
Dextrose 5%		7.0	8
To each 500 ml add	25 ml 50% dextrose		
	18 mmol NaCl		
	18 mmol KCl		
Dextrose 10%		7.0	8
Infuse Vamin Dextrose for 1 h, dextrose 5% for 1 h then dextrose 10% for 1 h			
Day 6+			
Intralipid 10%		1.5	20 (stop at 0600)
To each 100 ml add	Solivito 1.7 ml		
	Vitlipid Infant 3.3 ml		
	(to maximum of 4 ml/day)		
Vamin Dextrose		3.5	12
To each 100 ml add	11 ml Ped-el		
Dextrose 10%		6.5	12
To each 500 ml add	7 mmol NaCl		
	11 mmol KCl		
Infuse Vamin Dextrose for 1 h, then dextrose 10% for 1 h			

- Siting of drips may become impossible because of damage to veins
— Central lines are best placed using Silastic catheters
  - Use medical grade silastic tubing OD 0.025 in (Dow Corp. Medical Products, Michigan 48640, USA, ref. 602–105)
  - Prior to insertion measure distance to right nipple
  - Insert via 19G butterfly needle (extension tubing removed) in vein in antecubital fossa or scalp vein
  - Advance catheter slowly using no touch technique till distance to right nipple (roughly equivalent position to right atrium) is reached
  - Remove butterfly

Table 13.14 Ward-based parenteral nutrition regimen for children between 10 and 30 kg

Infusion fluid	Infusion rate (ml/kg/h)	Duration (h/day)
Days 1–2		
Intralipid* 10%	0.75	20 (stop at 0600)
Vamin Dextrose	2.0	8
To each 100 ml add 1.3 ml Addamel		
Dextrose 5%	4.0	16
To each 500 ml add 13 mmol NaCl		
17 mmol KCl		
Infuse Vamin Dextrose for 1 h, then dextrose 5% for 2 h		
Day 3+		
Intralipid* 10%	1.0	20 (stop at 0600)
Vamin Dextrose	2.5	12
To each 100 ml add 0.7 ml Addamel		
Dextrose 10%	4.0	12
To each 500 ml add 11 mmol NaCl		
20 mmol KCl		
Infuse Vamin Dextrose for 1 h, then dextrose 10% for 1 h		

* To the day's requirements of Intralipid add 5 ml Solivito
4 ml Vitlipid Infant.

Table 13.15 Ward-based parenteral nutrition regimen for children over 30 kg

Infusion fluid	Infusion rate (ml/kg/h)	Duration (h/day)
Days 1–2		
Intralipid* 10%	0.5	20 (stop at 0600)
Vamin Dextrose	2.0	8
To each 100 ml add 1.3 ml Addamel		
Dextrose 5%	2.0	16
To each 500 ml add 27 mmol NaCl		
34 mmol KCl		
Infuse Vamin Dextrose for 1 h, then dextrose 5% for 2 h		
Day 3+		
Intralipid* 10%	0.75	20 (stop at 0600)
Vamin Dextrose	2.0	12
To each 100 ml add 0.9 ml Addamel		
Dextrose 10%	2.0	12
To each 500 ml add 27 mmol NaCl		
42 mmol KCl		
Infuse Vamin Dextrose for 1 h, then dextrose 10% for 1 h		

* To the day's requirement of Intralipid add 5 ml Solivito
4 ml Vitlipid Infant.

- Thread needle guard on catheter
- Insert 25G long butterfly needle into catheter
- Cover needle tip with guard to prevent it 'cutting out'
- Check position of catheter tip radiologically using 0.6 ml warmed Hypaque

Table 13.16 Amounts of fluid, amino acids, fat, calories, sodium, potassium and Ped-el provided by ward-based parenteral nutrition regimen (amounts/kg/24 h)

Day of parenteral nutrition	Fluid (ml)	Amino acids (g)	Glucose (g)	Fat (g)	Non-N_2 energy kcal (kJ)	Na^+ (mmol)	K^+ (mmol)	Ped-el (ml)
(a) Less than 10 kg								
1	154	0.9	7	1	39 (164)	2.9	2.6	3.2
2–5	156	1.4	10	2	62 (260)	3.0	2.5	3.5
6	150	2.6	12	3	81 (340)	3.0	2.5	4.2
(b) 10–30 kg								Addamel
1–2	95	1.1	5	1.5	37 (153)	2.5	2.5	0.21
3	98	2.1	8	2	54 (227)	2.5	2.5	0.21
(c) >30 kg								
1–2	58	1.1	5	1	31 (130)	2.5	2.5	0.21
3	63	1.7	5	1.5	37 (153)	2.5	2.5	0.21

- Fix loops of catheter to the skin
- Larger catheters may be inserted via a 16 FG butterfly and threaded on a 23 FG butterfly
— If no suitable peripheral vein can be found, a catheter may be inserted into an external or internal jugular vein via a skin tunnel

Introduction of parenteral nutrition

— Before beginning parenteral nutrition, resuscitation with plasma or blood and correction of electrolyte and acid base disturbances should be undertaken
— Parenteral nutrition is introduced in a step-wise fashion over a period of at least a week to minimise metabolic complications (see pharmacy-based regimen for slower introduction in infants)
— Amounts delivered shown in Table 13.6

Monitoring

— Close liaison with a clinical chemistry department is essential
— Microanalytical methods also essential
— See Table 13.17 for details of monitoring

Complications

— See Table 13.18

Hyperlipidaemia

— Weekly lipid profile shows high triglyceride if clearance is inadequate

Table 13.17 Monitoring of patients receiving parenteral nutrition

Daily	3 times weekly	Weekly
Anthropometry		
Weight		Length
		Head circumference
Urine		
Glucose	Electrolytes	
Specific gravity		
Blood/plasma		
Dextrostix (or BM stix)		Glucose, albumin, ALT, alkaline phosphatase
(12 hourly for first week)		and gamma GT
Urea and electrolytes	Urea and electrolytes	Ca^{2+}, Mg^{2+}, P, Zn^{2+}, Cu^{2+}
(for one week)	(when stable)	
Plasma turbidity	Blood gas	Fe, transferrin, lipid profile, Hb, MCV, WBC,
		differential, platelet count

Table 13.18 Complications of parenteral nutrition

Biochemical

Hyperlipidaemia
Hypoglycaemia
Hyperglycaemia
Hyperosmolar dehydration
Hypophosphataemia (anaemia, thrombocytopenia, neutropenia, convulsions)
Essential fatty acid deficiency
Trace element deficiency (see Table 13.19)
Electrolyte disturbance
Hyperammonaemia
Acidosis
Hypoproteinaemia
Liver dysfunction

Technical

Extravasation
Thrombosis and embolus

Infection

Septicaemia
Other

Gastrointestinal

Pancreatic atrophy
Small intestine mucosal atrophy

Haematological

Anaemia

— Commonest in small for gestational age and preterm infants and with sepsis
— Slow increase and careful monitoring in small preterm infants
— Stop Intralipid infusion in uncontrolled sepsis because it is poorly metabolised
NB Monitor phosphate carefully (see hypophosphataemia below)
— Prevent essential fatty acid deficiency while Intralipid is not used by rubbing the skin with sunflower oil twice daily

Hypoglycaemia
— Malnourished infants particularly at risk
— Reactive hypoglycaemia occurs if drip is discontinued
  • Minimise delay in resiting of drips
  • During recovery phase out parenteral feeding slowly

Hyperglycaemia
— Impaired glucose tolerance may be a problem in:
  • Preterm infants
  • Postoperative period (48 h)
  • In sepsis
— Hyperglycaemia causes osmotic diuresis
— Monitor urine glucose daily
  • If >0.5% check blood sugar
  NB Low renal threshold may be cause of glycosuria
— If glucose tolerance is low (e.g. in preterms it may be as low as 8 g/kg/day) consider using insulin
  • If blood sugar >10 mmol/l
  • Soluble insulin 0.05 units/kg/h by IV infusion
  • May improve transport of glucose into cells without increasing metabolism resulting in intracellular overhydration and extracellular dehydration due to osmotic effect
  • Best avoided if possible

Hypophosphataemia
— Phosphate depletion commonly occurs when cells are released from mitotic arrest after introduction of nutrition
— Cells not undergoing mitosis become depleted resulting in
  • Anaemia
  • Neutrophil dysfunction
  • Platelet dysfunction
  • Neurological symptoms – weakness, convulsions and coma
— Supply extra phosphorus (0.5 mmol/kg/day) orally as K_2HPO_4 or via separate infusion in 5% dextrose

Hypocalcaemia
— Measure ionised Ca^{2+} if possible
— Correct plasma calcium for plasma albumin concentration
  • Corrected Ca^{2+} = measured Ca^{2+} + [(40 − measured albumin) × 0.019]
— If value persistently low after correction or symptoms occur increase calcium intake appropriately (e.g. 1 mmol/kg/day)
— Check Mg^{2+} after correction

Electrolyte disturbance
— Common only if abnormal losses continue from gastrointestinal or renal tracts
— Estimate losses by measurements of electrolytes in appropriate fluids, e.g. gastric aspirate, faeces, urine
— Hyponatraemia
  • Consider water overload (e.g. due to inappropriate ADH secretion) or Na^+ depletion
  • If inappropriate ADH (urine Na^+ > 20 mmol/l with hyponatraemia) treat by fluid restriction
  • Maintain urine Na^+:K^+ ratio at about 2:1
  • Urine Na^+:K^+ ratio <1:1 indicates significant sodium depletion
  • If depletion confirmed, increase daily intake by 1 mmol/kg/day until urine electrolytes are again appropriate

Hyperammonaemia
— May occur if amino acid intake recommendations are exceeded
— Preterm infants especially at risk
— Relatively uncommon with synthetic amino acid mixtures as compared with protein hydrolysates

Acidosis
— Rarely presents if alcohol and fructose are avoided as nutrients
— Vamin-Dextrose presents an acid load
— Sepsis may present as acidosis

Hypoproteinaemia
— Common in malnourished individuals
— Resultant fall in plasma oncotic pressure results in aldosterone and ADH secretion and water overload with oedema
— Treat if plasma albumin <25 g/l (20 g/l in the newborn)
— Give 1–3 g/kg of plasma protein as plasma protein fraction, plasma, or fresh frozen plasma

Liver dysfunction
— Jaundice is uncommon with parenteral nutrition
  • Commoner in surgical patients
  • Cholestatic type of jaundice
  • Early enteral feeding may prevent this complication
— Transient elevation of hepatic enzymes (ALT and gamma GT) may occur on reintroduction of enteral feeds

Infection
— Prevention involves scrupulous attention to detail
— Site infusions under conditions of maximum sterility
  • Spray insertion site with a povidine iodine spray
  • Cover site with porous adhesive tape
  • Change dressing only when contaminated or soaked (e.g. with sweat)
— Contamination of intravenous fluids

- Contamination undetectable to the naked eye until organism count $>10^9/l$
- Can occur through microscopic defects in containers, tubing, filters, etc.
- Minimise connections in giving system
- Avoid 3-way taps
- Protect air inlets with bacterial filters
- Change whole giving system daily
- Soak cannula connection in 0.5% chlorhexidine or spray with povidine iodine before changing
- Microaggregate filters may reduce thrombophlebitis and possibly infection but have to be placed above Intralipid inlet
- Do not use dedicated central lines for administration of drugs, blood products, etc. or for sampling

Management of pyrexial child
— Full septic screen and white blood count
  - Include pharyngeal secretions
  - Urine for *Candida* which is excreted in urine in septicaemia
  - Chest X-ray
  - Blood culture
— Start broad spectrum antibiotic therapy
— Stop amino acid and lipid infusion
— If fever not settled in 24 h and bacterial or fungal infection is suspected, remove central line
— Send tip for culture
— If no response to therapy in 48–72 h fungal infection must be considered likely and appropriate systemic therapy may be indicated

Gastrointestinal atrophy
— Cessation of enteral feeding results in atrophy of gastrointestinal mucosae and the pancreas even during parenteral nutrition
— If at all possible, a small amount of enteral feeding is continued though the minimum required to prevent atrophy is unknown

Trace element deficiency
— Requirements for trace elements may be high due to previous deficiency or growth spurt after introduction of IV feeding
— Clinical manifestations are protean (see Table 13.19)

REINTRODUCTION OF ENTERAL NUTRITION

— See Appendix B for constituents of feeds and additives
— A hypoallergenic diet is almost always used in infancy

Table 13.19 Clinical manifestations of trace element deficiency

Element	Signs of deficiency
Zinc	Perineal and periorbital dermatitis, diarrhoea, alopecia, paronychia, irritability, anorexia, immunodeficiency (mimics acrodermatitis enteropathica)
Copper	Anaemia, neutropenia, osteoporosis
Iodine	Goitrous hypothyroidism
Fluorine	Enamel hypoplasia, osteoporosis
Chromium	Impaired glucose tolerance, peripheral neuropathy
Selenium	Cardiomyopathy, myalgia
Manganese	Growth failure

Deficiencies of silicon, nickel, vanadium and tin have been reported in animals

— Pepti-Junior or Pregestimil
  • Complete formula including vitamins and minerals
  • No whole proteins or large peptides
  • Extra essential amino acids
  • No lactose or sucrose
  • Introduce as full strength at 1 ml/h and increase slowly
— Comminuted chicken-based diets are tolerated by some children who are intolerant of elemental diets
  • Allows independent variation of amounts of protein, carbohydrate and fat
  • See Table 13.20 for composition of complete feed made up as below
  • Requires additions including:
    – Carbohydrates as Maxijul
    – Fat as Calogen (Prosparol no longer made)
    – Minerals as Metabolic Mineral Mixture
    – Vitamins as Ketovite liquid and tablets
  • Very complex feed for home or hospital use
— Introduction of 'Chix' (comminuted chicken-based diet)
  • Initially 1 ml/h of 10% suspension
  • Increase concentration by 10% per day to 50% (full strength)
  • Add Metabolic Mineral Mixture at 1 g/100 ml when total daily volume of 100 ml is reached
    – Maximum 1.5 g/kg/day for infants less than 5 kg to overall maximum 8 g/day
  • Simultaneously withdraw Ped-el from parenteral regimen
  • Add Ketovite liquid (5 ml/day) and tablets (3/day) and withdraw parenteral vitamin supplements
  • Add carbohydrate as Maxijul 1 g/100 ml increasing by 1 g/100 ml daily to maximum of 8–12 g/100 ml monitoring stool for carbohydrate

Table 13.20 Amounts of fluid, protein, carbohydrate, fat, calories, Na^+, K^+, Ca^{2+}, Mg^{2+}, P and Fe^{3+} provided by full strength comminuted chicken feed (amounts/kg/day)

	Comminuted chicken 50%	Maxijul	Calogen	Metabolic mineral mix	Total
Fluid (ml)	200	–	10	–	210
Protein (g)	7.5	–	–	–	7.5
Carbohydrate (g)	–	20	–	–	20
Fat (g)	2.5–4	–	5	–	7.5–9
Non-N_2 kcal	23–36	80	45	–	148–161
(kJ)	(97–151)	(336)	(189)	–	(622–676)
Na^+ (mmol)	0.4	2	0.07	2.6	5.1
K^+ (mmol)	1.3	0.2	–	3.2	4.7
Ca^{2+} (mmol)	0.2	–	–	3.1	3.3
Mg^{2+} (mmol)	0.3	–	–	0.6	0.9
P (mmol)	1.5	–	–	2.9	4.4
Fe^{3+} (mmol/mg)	(0.007)	–	–	(0.012)	(0.02)
	0.04	–	–	0.7	0.79

- Add fat as an emulsion of long-chain fat (Calogen) commencing at 1 ml (0.5 g)/100 ml and increasing by 1 ml/100 ml daily to maximum of 8 ml/100 ml
- Increase total volume of feed by 5–20% of total requirement per day depending on tolerance

NB Small infants may not tolerate full intake of comminuted chicken without raised blood urea

- See Figure 5.2 for reintroduction of other feeds
- Consider transfer to other complete formula mild substitute before discharge by gradual substitution in total daily volume

FURTHER TREATMENT OF MALNOURISHED INFANTS ESTABLISHED ON ORAL FEEDS

— Values given for actual not 'expected weight'
— Require increased energy intake as tolerated. 130–220 kcal (540–900 kJ) kg/day
— Increased protein intake is often desirable
  - Under 6 months 3–6 g/kg/day
  - Over a year 10 g/kg/day (maximum)
— To attain above intake large volumes of feeds may be convenient
  - 180–220 ml/kg/day maximum in preterm infants
  - 200–300 ml/kg/day in older infants achieved over a period of gradual increase
— Ensure adequate intake of electrolytes, calcium, vitamins and trace elements

NUTRITION OF PRETERM INFANTS

— Enteral, parenteral/enteral or parenteral according to gastro-intestinal function
— Specialised formulae available for preterm infants
  • Relatively high protein to try to reproduce intrauterine growth
  • Na^+ content also increased to allow for increased renal Na^+ loss in preterm
  • Energy content increased to allow decreased volume. (Necrotising enterocolitis and persistent patent ductus arteriosus have been related to high fluid intake)
— Expressed breast milk nutritionally suboptimal and requires modification
  • Can be supplemented with Na^+
  • Fortification with Pepti-Junior or Pregestimil (3% in breast milk) can provide increased calories and nitrogen without increasing lactose or adding protein of non-human origin
  • Hind milk may be richer
— Vitamin supplements necessary (especially E and D)

NUTRITIONAL PROBLEMS OF THE NEONATE AFTER MAJOR SURGERY

— Special problems likely to be encountered in these patients are summarised in Table 13.21
— Early introduction of enteral feeding is essential in neonatal surgical patients to
  • Stimulate adaptation of remaining bowel
  • Prevent gastrointestinal atrophy associated with withholding enteral nutrition
  • Prevent cholestasis

Short gut syndrome

— Short gut syndrome may arise following massive resections, e.g. for volvulus due to malrotation, multiple small bowel atresias
— Severe watery diarrhoea supervenes once ileus has resolved
— Management is as for protracted diarrhoea (p. 43)
— Modular diet based on comminuted chicken can be successfully introduced in patients in whom elemental diets are not tolerated
— Cholestyramine may help bile acid induced diarrhoea

Table 13.21 Nutritional problems in the surgical neonate

Problem	Causes	Prevention
Oedema	Inappropriate ADH secretion	Restrict fluid intake to one-third requirements for 24 h postop. Increase over 3 days to full requirement
	Hypoproteinaemia	Monitor serum albumin weekly
	Mg^{2+} deficiency, e.g. due to diuretics	Monitor Mg^{2+}
Na^+ depletion	Inadequate replacement of GI losses, diuretics. NB Hyponatraemia due to inappropriate ADH secretion is not Na^+ depletion	Monitor urine and plasma Na^+ and K^+, maintaining urinary Na^+ at 20–40 mmol/l and Na^+/K^+ ratio at about 2:1
K^+ depletion	As for Na^+ depletion. NB Na^+ depletion causes increased urinary K^+ losses	Monitor urine and plasma K^+ Maintain urinary K^+ at 10–20 mmol/l
Hypophosphataemia	Increased requirement during catch-up growth following malnutrition	Monitor plasma phosphorus
Lactose intolerance	Resection of jejunum. Damage due to necrotising enterocolitis	Low lactose diet (see text)

Lactose intolerance

— Lactose intolerance common
— Presents as watery diarrhoea containing reducing substances (>0.5% on stool Clinitest)
— Associated with Na^+ depletion (urinary Na^+ concentration <10 mmol/litre) and poor growth/weight loss
— Change to lactose-free feed (e.g. Pregestimil)
— Introduce slowly as full strength feed (1 ml per hour) and increase 6–24-hourly according to tolerance
— Administer by nasogastric tube, preferably as a continuous infusion
— A few infants also intolerant of the carbohydrate in Pregestimil (glucose polymer) and develop diarrhoea
  NB Pepti-Junior has lower carbohydrate content
— A trial of a modular feed based on comminuted chicken (Cow and Gate) ('Chix') then indicated (see above)
— Substitute Maxijul (glucose polymer) as sole carbohydrate, with 7% Maxijul/3% sucrose mixture
— Lactose-containing formula may be introduced when infant thriving

ENTERAL NUTRITION IN INFANCY AND CHILDHOOD

Indications

— Crohn's disease (induction of remission)
— Cystic fibrosis*

— Short gut
— Advanced cirrhosis*
— Postoperative newborn
— Severe congenital heart disease*
— Chronic renal failure*
— Protracted diarrhoea
— Cerebral palsy*
— Anorexia nervosa
— Malignancy*

*Results in improved growth but not necessarily associated with improved prognosis overall

Type of feed
— Advice of paediatric dietitian essential
— Elemental diet (amino acids, glucose polymer and fat) usually given in Crohn's disease (e.g. Elemental 028)
— Hydrolysed protein/glucose polymer-based feed (e.g. Flexical; Mead Johnson)
— Hydrolysed whey or casein/glucose polymer-based feed, or comminuted chicken-based diet usually given in protracted diarrhoea and short gut
— A whole protein-based feed usually suitable for other indications (e.g. Fortison Paediatric, Isocal)

Routes of administration
Nasogastric tube
— Soft Silastic or polyethylene tube (e.g. 'Silk'; Merck) comfortable and requires less frequent changing (every few months) than PVC tubes (changed every 7–10 days)
— Softer tubes require guide wire for insertion
Nasojejunal tube
— Indicated only for gastroparesis
— Difficult to site and retain in position
— Diarrhoea more likely than with nasogastric administration, particularly when hyperosmolar feeds used
Jejunostomy tube
— Rarely indicated
  • Used for long-term feeding
  • In patients with severe gastroparesis associated with intractable gastrooesophageal reflux and pulmonary aspiration
  • (Usually following surgery for oesophageal atresia/tracheo-oesophageal fistula)
— Requires surgical insertion
— Diarrhoea with hyperosmolar feeds and rapid transit
Technique of administration
— Less diarrhoea with continuous infusion
— In protracted diarrhoea nutrient balances better with continuous feeding than with bolus administration

— Constant infusion pump necessary to enable accurate administration
— Pump should run from mains and from rechargeable battery to provide patient mobility
— Small portable pumps available for home enteral feeding
— When given as supplement, overnight infusion often possible

Complications

— With the exception of nocturia, complications are rare and preventable
— Nocturia
— Osmotic diarrhoea
— Feeling of fullness and vomiting (therefore introduce over 2–3 days)
— Gastro-oesophageal reflux + pulmonary aspiration
— Rhinorrhoea secondary to nasogastric tube
— Obesity
— Nutrient imbalances from administration of inappropriate feeds

14 CERTAIN INVESTIGATION PROTOCOLS

Continuous ambulatory intraoesophageal pH monitoring

— The current 'gold standard' for the detection and quantification of gastrooesophageal acid reflux
— Calibrate the recorder using buffers of known pH
— Place the tip of the probe at a known distance above the gastro-oesophageal sphincter
  • Calculated from manometry study if done or
  • Positioned opposite T9 or T10 on radiographic screening
— Record pH for at least 20 h
— Analyse the record with reference to a contemporary diary of
  • Meal times
  • Sleep/wake state
  • Upright/supine position
  • Symptoms experienced
— Computer programmes are available to calculate
  • Percent time with pH below 4
  • Total
  • Upright
  • Supine
  • Number of reflux episodes per 24 h
  • Number of reflux episodes lasting >5 minutes per 24 h
  • Duration of longest reflux episode
— A reflux episode is generally defined as a fall below pH 4 for >20 seconds
— Age related normal values are available in the literature

Combined jejunal biopsy pancreatic function test

— NB These tests should only be done after supervised experience. The following are hints, not instructions

Equipment
— Equipment we use and have found reliable
— Modified Crosby–Kugler jejunal biopsy capsule (Figure 14.1)
  • Spring integral with knife blade

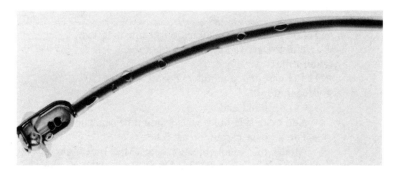

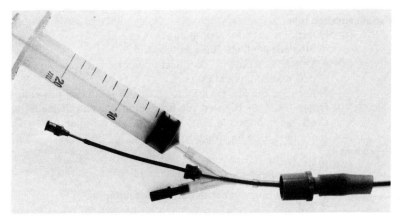

Figure 14.1 Modified Crosby–Kugler jejunal biopsy needle

- • External 'clip' holds capsule reliably together
- • Adult capsule in children over 30 kg
- • Single (large hole) capsule in children over 12 kg
- • Single small hole or, better, the double hole (TC Components Limited, 44 Uxbridge Road, Hampton, Middx TW12 3AD) in infants under 12 kg
— 'Firing' tube
  - • Kifa (red)
    - – Tough – lasts many biopsies
    - – Radio-opaque
    - – Semirigid
    - – Firm seal with capsule
  - • Portex (800/023/150)
    - – Flexible – passes easily round pyloric canal/duodenal cap in small infants
    - – Requires protection from teeth (see below)
    - – Outer tube can be used to vary tension and rigidity

— Guide wire
- Teflon coated (e.g. Selflex, 0.889 mm × 150 cm)
- Useful to vary rigidity of flexible tube
— Outer tube
- 12 FG nasoduodenal tube (Portex 400/100/120)
- Preparation:
  - Cut off blind end
  - Add extra side holes which should be small and numerous
  - Thread over capsule firing tube
  - Attach to a dual injection site (MacGraw Labs V5600, Irvine, California 92705, USA; Boots UK) as shown in Figure 14.1

Use of combined tube
— Outer tube used for aspiration
- Stomach contents during intubation
- Duodenal contents for microbiology, bile salt analysis, pancreatic function test
— Outer tube can also be used for giving drugs during procedure
— Outer tube can be used for instillation of contrast media to check tube position in cases of doubt (e.g. malrotation)
— Inner tube used for firing capsule **only**

Procedure
— Fast
- Overnight in children
- 4–6 h in infants or malnourished children
— Sedation
- Trimeprazine 4–5 mg/kg 1 to 2 hours before procedure in toddlers 6 months to 4 years
- In small infants and older children and as an addition in toddlers use Diazepam
  - Diazemuls is a solution in Intralipid and is pain-free on intravenous injection
  - 0.5 mg/kg to (5–10 mg maximum) is initial dose
  - Sufficient to cause muscle relaxation and ptosis is necessary for adequate sedation
  - Has the advantage of producing amnesia
— Protect biopsy tube and operator's fingers from teeth
- Use an oral nasal tracheal tube (Portex 100/111/090) or similar wide-bore tube round the outside of the capsule tubes (Figure 14.1)
— If the capsule is placed over the back of the tongue by a finger and gently advanced it will be swallowed
— Too rapid pushing down the oesophagus causes gagging
— Turn patient on to the right side as the capsule reaches the stomach thus directing it toward the pylorus
— Turn the patient back into the supine position when it is estimated tube is near pylorus as pyloric canal runs posteriorly

— If using image intensifier screening capsule appears fore-shortened as it turns posteriorly adjacent to the right side of the vertebrae

— Delayed passage through the pylorus may be aided by Metoclopromide 0.3 mg/kg IV

— Avoid loops of tube in stomach by only advancing tube as capsule progresses

— If screening do not 'watch' capsule but rather observe intermittently with very short episodes of screening

— If in doubt as to whether tube is coiled in stomach or is in duodenum
  • Observe in full lateral when tube passes into right paravertebral gully as it passes through the duodenal cap

— Delay at junction of 2nd and 3rd parts of duodenum may be due to pressure from coeliac axis
  • Turning the patient to prone will overcome this

— Pass tube till capsule is at duodenojejunal flexure

Pancreatic function test

— Tape tube to cheek

— Maintain stomach empty by means of nasogastric tube passed now rather than earlier

— Aspirate fasting juice via outer tube and send for
  • Bicarbonate assay
  • Pancreatic enzyme assays
  • Bile salt analysis
  • Microbiology

— Collect anaerobically and process immediately, or put straight in anaerobic transport medium and freeze on solid carbon dioxide

— Fresh unfrozen specimen for *Giardia* by direct microscopy

— Use gastric function pump for aspiration if this is available
  • e.g. United Analysts Ltd, East Boldon, Tyne and Wear, UK
  • Volume of recovery is much enhanced compared with intermittent syringe suction

— Hormonal stimulation (maximal response)
  • 2 u/kg IV (after test doses) of cholecystokinin pancreozymin and secretin and collect juice for 30 minutes
  NB Add equal volume 5% dextrose in 50/50 quantity before storing if enzyme analysis is delayed and store at $-20°C$
  • See Table 14.1 for normal values

— Test meal stimulation (physiological response)
  • Using modified Lundh meal (glucose, corn oil) and comminuted chicken each at 4 g/100 ml in a dose of 30 ml/kg to a maximum of 240 ml)
  • Collect juice over 2 h
  • Stable enzyme activity without dextrose
  • Nasogastric tube used to give meal not to empty stomach
  • Bicarbonate cannot be assayed
  • See Table 14.1

Table 14.1 Activities of pancreatic enzymes, bicarbonate and total bile salt concentrations in control[1] children following various methods of pancreaticobiliary stimulation.

	Trypsin[2] (μEq/min/ml)			Lipase[3] (μEq/min/ml)			Amylase[4] (units/ml)			Bicarbonate[5] (mmol/l)			Total bile salts[6] (mmol/l)		
	n	Mean	Range	n	Mean	Range	n	Mean	Range	n	Mean	Range	n	Mean	Range
Test meal	13	43	19–83	13	768	270–1920	–	–	–	–	–	–	9	6.8	2.7–16.0
Post-cholecystokinin and secretin	21	56	29–106	21	1195	696–2664	20	185	30–401	6	59	36–70	13	17.3	6.2–32.0
Post-cholecystokinin	9	71	48–108	10	1040	363–1930	8	282	119–525	–	–	–	9	37.1	17.7–54.7

[1] Children (aged 9 months to 16 years) with suspected malabsorption were proven to be normal following intensive investigation.
[2] Titrimetic assay using p-tosyl arginine methyl ester as substrate.
[3] Titrimetic assay.
[4] Amylochrome kit supplied by Roche Products Ltd.
[5] Colorimetric assay using cresol red.
[6] Enzymatic method.

Jejunal biopsy

— Even if not performing pancreatic function test, a duodenal aspirate for microbiology may be obtained using outer tube
— Rinse firing tube with 5 ml of normal saline
— Empty firing tube by 5 ml of air
— Attach 20 ml syringe
— Pull gently until suction is established by mucosa over holes in capsule
— Pull hard to 20 ml to fire capsule
— Too rapid initial suction sometimes results in the capsule firing on mucus or an inadequate specimen
— Remove capsule and open
— Gently ease mucosal sample(s) from capsule and spread shiny, concave side uppermost on a fingertip (mucosa downwards)
— Lift off finger tip by applying a piece of dry card. Black card gives good visualisation under dissecting microscope

Faecal fat excretion

— Commonly called but rarely is a 'fat balance'
— Rarely indicated because gives no diagnostic information
— Dietary fat must be adequate to stress absorptive system
  • Infants 5 g/kg/day
  • 1–5 years 40–50 g/day
  • 6–12 years 50–80 g/day
  • Adults 100 g/day
— Ensure regular bowel movement before starting tests
— Use carmine and/or Edecol blue markers at beginning (time zero) and end (time zero + 72 hours) of study
— Analyse stools including first marked stool and discarding first stool containing second marker and subsequent stools
— At all ages >5 g/day excretion is abnormal
— Coefficients of absorption vary with age
  • Preterm infant   >60% absorption
  • Term infant   >80% absorption
  • 1–6 months   >85% absorption
  • 6 m to 12 y   >90% absorption
  • <12 y   >95% absorption

Gastric acid secretion test

— Fasting pH>4 suggests achlorhydria or indicates adequate H_2 antagonist therapy
— Gastric acid secretion must be measured to test function
  • Overnight fast (shorter in infants)
  • Pass nasogastric tube
  • Empty stomach and discard contents

- Basal acid output (BAO) estimated by collection of four 15-minute samples
- Give intravenous pentagastrin (6 μg/kg)
- Collect eight 15-minute samples for analysis
- Maximum acid output (MAO) is rate of acid secretion in first hour
- Peak acid output (PAO) is sum of highest two consecutive 15-minute outputs × 2, i.e. mmol/h
- Acid output measured in laboratory as titratable acidity with 0.1 M sodium hydroxide to pH 7
— Normal values close to those of adults on a body-weight basis
— In Zollinger–Ellison syndrome, BAO is very high but little increase with pentagastrin. Gastrin levels very high in fasting blood

Carbohydrate absorption

— Carbohydrate is present in the fluid phase
  - Stool must be collected on plastic and separate from urine
  - Liquid phase must be tested
— Digestion by enzymes and bacteria continues after stool is passed
  - Test stools immediately
  - If transferred to laboratory freeze at −20°C
— pH of stool is an unreliable indicator of carbohydrate malabsorption
— Dilute 5 drops of stool fluid with 10 drops of water and add 1 Clinitest (Ames) tablet
NB If testing for sucrose, boil first with dilute HCl to hydrolyse
— Read as urine
— More than 0.5% reducing substances suggests carbohydrate malabsorption
— Note: normal breast-fed babies often have increased reducing substances due to rapid transit and breast milk oligosaccharides
— Confirm abnormal findings by thin-layer chromatography

Carbohydrate challenge

— Load method: 1 g sugar under investigation/kg (+ Carmine marker) given to fasting patient followed by normal diet after 2 hours
  - Test loose (marked) stools with Clinitest and send for chromatography
— Introduction method: introduce 1% carbohydrate and increase daily by 1% to total of 4–6%
  - Test any watery stools as above

B$_{12}$ absorption – Schilling test

Phase 1

— Administration of test
  - During a 4-h fast
  - At 2 h give [^{57}Co]B$_{12}$ 0.5 μCi (18 kBq) orally
  - At 4 h give cold B$_{12}$ 1 mg by intramuscular injection
  - Collect all urine for 24 h
  - Measure [^{57}Co]B$_{12}$ in urine collected
— Interpretation
  - >10% of administered dose in urine is a normal result
  - <10% indicates malabsorption but not cause

Phase 2

— Administration
— Repeat as above but giving intrinsic factor with the [^{57}Co]B$_{12}$ orally
— Interpretation
  - >10% on this phase and <10% on phase 1 confirms intrinsic factor deficiency
  - <10% in both phases confirms malabsorption but not intrinsic factor deficiency and suggests terminal ileal disease

APPENDIX A VITAMIN AND MINERAL REQUIREMENTS OF INFANTS AND CHILDREN

Vitamin requirements of infants and children*

	Infants		Children			Boys		Girls	
	0–6 m	6–12 m	1–3 y	4–6 y	7–10 y	11–14 y	15–17 y	11–14 y	15–17 y
Ascorbic acid (C) (mg)	20	20	20	20	20	25	30	25	30
Thiamin (B$_1$) (mg)	0.3	0.5	0.5	0.7	0.9	1.1	1.2	0.9	0.9
Nicotinic acid (niacin) (mg)	5	7	7	10	14	16	19	16	19
Riboflavin (B$_2$) (mg)	0.4	0.6	0.6	0.9	1.2	1.4	1.7	1.4	1.7
Pyridoxine (B$_6$) (mg)	0.4	0.6	0.7	0.9	1.2	1.5	1.5	1.5	1.5
Folic acid (µg)	50	50	100	150	200	300	300	300	300
Cyanocobalamin (B$_{12}$) (µg)	0.3	0.5	1.0	1.5	2.0	3.0	3.0	3.0	3.0
Retinol (A) (µg)	450	450	300	400	575	725	750	725	750
Cholecalciferol (D) (µg)	7.5	10	10	†	†	†	†	†	†
Tocopherol (E) (iu)	4	5	7	9	10	12	15	12	12

* Data derived primarily from British Recommended Daily Allowances, but some data from USA where appropriate.
† Beyond 4 years requirements may be supplied by sufficient exposure to sunlight.

Mineral requirements of infants and children

		Infants		Children			Boys		Girls	
		0–6 m	6–12 m	1–3 y	4–6 y	7–10 y	11–14 y	15–17 y	11–14 y	15–17 y
Calcium	(mg)	360	540	800	800	800	1200	1200	1200	1200
	(mmol)	18	27	40	40	40	60	60	60	60
Magnesium	(mg)	60	70	150	200	200	350	400	300	300
	(mmol)	5	6	12	17	1	30	32	25	25
Phosphate	(mg)	240	400	800	800	800	1200	1200	1200	1200
	(mmol)	3	5	10	10	10	15	15	15	15
Iodine	(mg)	35	45	60	80	110	130	150	115	115
Iron	(mg)	10	15	15	10	10	18	18	18	18
Zinc	(mg)	3	5	10	10	10	15	15	15	15

APPENDIX B SPECIAL NUTRITIONAL SUPPLEMENTS AND FEEDS

Dietary products and suggested feeds for specific purposes in infants

Normal term infant
- Mother's breast milk
- 'Standard' infant formula (humanised cow's milk based)

Preterm infant
- Mother's fresh expressed breast milk (see p. 00)
- Preterm formulae of most manufacturers

Atopic family history
- Mother's breast milk if at all possible
- If cow's milk protein-free diet is required, OsterSoy, Formula S, Isomil or Wysoy are the cheapest complete formula cow's milk-free feeds
- Goat's milk is often chosen by parents but requires dilution and addition of CHO and vitamins
- Other protein sensitivity may develop. Some suggest whole protein-free (see below)

Vegetarian
- Formula S and OsterSoy are a complete formula milk with no animal products
  - Therefore acceptable to vegans

Cow's milk protein-free
- See above under Atopic family history

Whole protein-free (e.g. protracted diarrhoea/postsurgical)
- Pepti-Junior or Pregestimil are simplest complete formula
  - Pepti-Junior contains added carnitine
- Other similar feeds include Alfare and Prejomin
- Nutramigen is similar to Pregestimil without MCT
- Comminuted chicken may be indicated in exceptional circumstances (whole chicken protein)
- Also Pepdite 0–2, Pepdite 0–2 MCT and Neocate
  - Pepdite milks are beef/soy protein hydrolysates
  - Neocate contains ammino acids rather than peptides

Lactose-free (lactose intolerance/galactosaemia)
- OsterSoy, Formula S and Wysoy are the cheapest
- Others are expensive for this purpose

Lactose–galactose-free
> — Galactomin 17 for use in galactosaemia and galactokinase deficiency
> > • Reformulated as complete formula in 1990

Glucose–galactose-free
> — Fructose formula Galactomin 19
> > • Reformulated as complete formula in 1991

Monosaccharide intolerance (e.g. postsurgery/postgastroenteritis)
> — Fructose formula Galactomin 19 is often helpful in glucose intolerance

Sucrose intolerance/fructosaemia
> — Any standard cow's milk infant formula avoiding addition of common sugar
> NB Sucrose-free medicines

Protracted diarrhoea
> — See under Whole Protein-Free and see p. 43

Intestinal lymphangiectasia
> — Portagen
> NB Not a 'humanised' formula
> — MCT Pepdite 0–2

Details of formulae which we frequently use for infants

> — Suitable for complete nutrition of infants except as stated
> — Composition given as
> > • Main ingredients in g/100 ml of feed
> > • Energy (total) in kcals (kJ) per 100 ml of feed

Comminuted chicken meat (Cow & Gate)
> > • See text for details
> > • Though a whole protein feed it appears to be hypoallergenic, has a low osmolality and is well tolerated
> > • Main advantage is flexibility as it is made from individual ingredients
> > • Main disadvantage is complexity

Formula S soya food (Cow & Gate) 12.5% solution
> > • Cheap, cow's milk-free, low disaccharide, lactose-free
> > • Available 'over the counter'
> > > – Soy isolate and methionine   2.0
> > > – Glucose syrup solids   6.8
> > > – Vegetable oil   3.0
> > > – Energy   60 (252)

Galactomin Formula 17 (Cow & Gate) 13.1% solution
> > • Now a complete formula
> > • Insignificant traces of lactose (<13 mg/100 ml)
> > • Low osmolality (210 mmol/l)
> > > – Casein (washed)   1.9
> > > – Glucose syrup solids   7.4

      – Vegetable oils   3.4
      – Energy   66 (280)

Galactomin Fructose Formula 19 (Cow & Gate) 13.1% solution
- Now a complete formula
- High osmolality (407 mmol/l)
  - Casein (washed)   1.9
  - Fructose   6.4
  - Vegetable oils   4.0
  - Energy   67 (280)

OsterSoy (Farley) 13.3%
- Available over the counter
- Cheap, cow's milk-free, vegetarian and vegan acceptable, low disaccharide, lactose-free
  - Soy isolate and methionine   2.0
  - Glucose syrup solids   7.0
  - Vegetable oil   3.8
  - Energy   70 (294)

Pepti-Junior (Cow & Gate) 13.1% solution
- Similar to Pregestimil
- Added carnitine
- Lower carbohydrate (and higher fat)
- Low osmolality
- Palatable
  - Hydrolysed whey   2.0
  - Corn syrup   7.1
  - MCT and corn oil   3.7
  - Energy   66 (280)

Portagen Lactose-Free Formula (Mead Johnson) 15% solution
- Not a modified formula so unsuitable under 6 months
  - Sodium caseinate   2.5
  - Corn syrup solids   8.2
  - MCT and corn oil   3.4
  - Energy   70 (296)

Pregestimil (Mead Johnson) 15% solution
- Whole protein free non-antigenic food
- Disaccharide free
  - Hydrolysed casein   1.9
  - Corn syrup solids and starch 9.1
  - MCT and corn oil   2.7
  - Energy   60 (252)

Wysoy (Wyeth) 13.5% solution
- Cheap, milk-free, lactose-free, nutritionally adequate diet
- Available 'over the counter'
  - Soy isolate and methionine   2.0
  - Sucrose and corn syrup solids 6.9
  - Vegetable fats   3.6
  - Energy   67 (280)

Milks not detailed and reason

Product	Company	
AL 110	Nestlé	Not complete or modified formula
Granolac	Granose	Superseded on cost grounds
MCT (1) Milk	Cow & Gate	Not complete or modified formula
Nutramigen	Mead Johnson	Not modified
Prosobee Liquid	Mead Johnson	As for Granolac
Prosobee Powder	Mead Johnson	As for Granolac
Trisorbon	BDH	Not modified formula. Not cow's milk protein-free

Additives useful in gastroenterology

Protein sources

Casilan (Farley Glaxo)
- Washed casein
- Not a complete food
- Trace of lactose

Super Soluble Maxipro HBV (Scientific Hospital Supplies)
- Dialysed whey protein
- Not a complete food

Protifar (Cow & Gate)
- Skimmed milk protein
- Clinically nil lactose
- Not a complete food

Albumaid Complete (Scientific Hospital Supplies)
- Hydrolysed beef serum
- Not a complete food

Carbohydrate sources (partially hydrolysed starch)

Caloreen (Roussel)
- <1.8 mmol sodium
- <0.3 mmol potassium
- 384 kcal (1606 kJ)   per 100 g

Polycal (Cow & Gate)
- 2.2 mmol sodium
- 1.3 mmol potassium
- 330 kcal (1588 kJ)   per 100 g

Super Soluble Maxijul (Scientific Hospital Supplies)
- 2.0 mmol sodium
- 0.1 mmol potassium
- 360 kcal (1505 kJ)   per 100 g

LE Maxijul (Scientific Hospital Supplies) (low electrolyte)
- 0.01 mmol sodium
- 0.61 mmol potassium
- 360 kcal (1505 kJ)   per 100 g

Fat sources (essentially carbohydrate and protein-free)

MCT oil (Mead Johnson, Cow & Gate, Scientific Hospital Services)
- Triglycerides of C8 and C10
- Saturated fatty acids
- Brands vary slightly in composition of fatty acids
- Free of essential fatty acids
- 100 g fat/110 ml
- 830 kcal (3500 kJ)   per 100 g

Liquigen (Scientific Hospital Supplies)
- MCT emulsion (52%)
- 52 g MCT fat/100 ml
- 400 kcal (1700 kJ)   per 100 g

Calogen (Scientific Hospital Supplies)
- 50% arachis oil emulsion in water
- Long chain fatty acids and essential fatty acids
- 50 g fat/100 ml
- 450 kcal (1880 kJ)   per 100 g

Safflower oil, sunflower oil, corn oil, soy oil
- Oils rich in essential fatty acids
- Vary in content according to type of oil
- 100 g fat/100 ml
- 900 kcal (3700 kJ)   per 100 g

Fat and carbohydrate sources

Duocal (Scientific Hospital Supplies) (liquid or powder)
- 23 g carbohydrate/100 ml
- 7.1 g fat/100 ml (30% as MCT)
- 150 kcal/100 ml
- May require dilution for under 5 years

Products for older children

Useful dietary substitutes

NB Though 'complete' formulae with added minerals and vitamins, they are generally not suitable for use as sole nutrition in infants and may need to be modified for younger children

Composition given as
- Main ingredients in g/100 ml of feed
- Energy (non-nitrogen) in kcals (kJ)
- Osmolality of made up feed in mmol/kg

Whole protein feeds

Fortison Paediatric (Cow & Gate) undiluted
- Low osmolality
- Reasonably palatable
- Suitable for young children
  - Caseinate protein   2.7
  - Maltodextrin   12.0

– Vegetable oil	4.5
– Non-N$_2$ energy	101 (425)
– Osmolality	233

Other similar whole protein feeds
- Fortison, Fortison Plus (1.5 kcal/ml), Clinifeed iso, Clinifeed Favour, Liquisorb, Nutrauxil, Osmolite, Paediasure

Peptide feeds

Pepdite 2+ (Scientific Hospital Supplies) 20% solution
- Hydrolysed meat and soya peptides and amino acids 2.8
- Maltodextrin (corn origin) 12.6
- Vegetable oils 3.6
- Non-N$_2$ energy 79 (330)
- Osomolality 288

Elemental feeds

Elemental 028 (Scientific Hospital Supplies)
- Amino acids 2.8
- Protein equivalent 1.8
- Maltodextrin 13.6
- Vegetable oil 1.2
- Non-N$_2$ energy 63 (263)
- Osmolality 440

Cow's milk substitutes

Product	Company	Description
Plamil	Plantmilk	Plant food very low in carbohydrate and calcium. Soya based. Not a complete feed
Granogen	Granose	Soya food powder. Not a complete feed
Soy Bean Milk	Stona	Soya food powder. Not a complete feed
Pareve-Mate (Kosher)	Carnation	Jewish Coffee-Mate which is milk-free. Of no nutritional value. A 'convenience food'
Coffee-Mate	Carnation	Coffee creamer. Not complete food. Contains casein, dried glucose syrup, vegetable fat
Compliment	Cadbury	Coffee creamer. Not complete food. Contains casein, dried glucose syrup, vegetable fat
Gold	St Ivel	Soy food powder. Not a complete food but has added calcium

Lactase treated milks

Product	Company	Description
Digestelact	Hunter Valley Sharpe, Australia	Powdered lactase treated milk Contains galactose and glucose with approximately 2% lactose. Contains cow's milk protein
Lactalac	Cooperative Condensfabriek 'Friesland', Leeuwarden Holland	Similar to above

Lactase enzyme preparations

Product	Company	Description
Lactaid	Sugarlo, USA Granose Food, UK	Lactase enzyme sachets for reducing milk lactose
Maxilact	Gist Brocades, Industrial Foods Division, Delft, Holland	Similar to above

APPENDIX C
CONVERSIONS ETC.

Energy

Protein	1 g gives 17 kJ (4 Cals)
Fat	1 g gives 37 kJ (9 Cals)
MCT fat	1 g gives 34 kJ (8 Cals)
Carbohydrate	1 g gives 16 kJ (4 Cals)

Kilocalories (Cals) to kilojoules (kJ) $\times$ 4.184
Kilocalories (Cals) to megajoules (MJ) $\times$ 4.184 $\times 10^{-3}$

Concentrations

% = g/100 ml
mg to mmol divide by mol.wt
mg/100 ml to mmol/l divide by mol.wt and multiply by 10
mEq to mmol divide by valency

Molecular weights

Sodium	Na^+	23
Potassium	K^+	39.1
Calcium	Ca^{2+}	40.1
Magnesium	Mg^{2+}	24.3
Iron	Fe^{3+}	55.8
Zinc	Zn^{2+}	65.4
Copper	Cu^{2+}	63.5
Chloride	Cl^-	35.5
Bicarbonate	HCO_3^-	61
Phosphorus	P	31
Phosphate	PO_4^-	95
Lactate		89
Acetate		59
Sulphate	SO_4^-	96

Formula weights and mmol/g

		Mol.wt	mmol/g
Sodium chloride	NaCl	58.5	17.1
Sodium bicarbonate	NaHCO$_3$	84	11.9
Potassium chloride	KCl	74.6	13.4
Dipotassium hydrogen phosphate (anhydrous)	K$_2$HPO$_4$	174.1	5.7
Potassium dihydrogen phosphate	KH$_2$PO$_4$	136	7.4
Calcium chloride (anhydrous)	CaCl$_2$	111	9.0
Calcium lactate	Ca(CH$_3$CH(OH)COO)$_2$	218.1	4.6
Calcium gluconate	Ca(HO.CH$_2$(CHOH)$_4$COO)$_2$H$_2$O	448.4	2.2
Magnesium chloride	MgCl$_2$.6H$_2$O	203.3	4.9
Magnesium sulphate	MgSO$_4$7H$_2$O	246.5	4.1
Zinc acetate	Zn(CH$_3$COO)$_2$2H$_2$O	219.5	4.6
Zinc sulphate	ZnSO$_4$	161.4	6.2
Copper acetate	Cu(CH$_3$COO)$_2$H$_2$O	199.5	5.0
Copper sulphate	CuSO$_4$5H$_2$O	249.7	4.0

Solute load

NB Protein contributes 4 mosmol/kg for each gram

INDEX